Quellen und Forschungen zur Südsee

Reihe B: Forschungen

Herausgegeben von
Hermann Joseph Hiery

Band 1

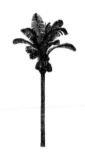

2002
Harrassowitz Verlag · Wiesbaden

Margrit Davies

Public Health and Colonialism

The Case of German New Guinea
1884–1914

2002

Harrassowitz Verlag · Wiesbaden

Umschlagabbildung: Marinestabsarzt Dr. Emil Stephan (sitzend) behandelt mit Hilfe des
Ethnologen Otto Schlaginhaufen einen einheimischen Patienten am Muliamabach
(Südost-Neumecklenburg), 1908.
Museum für Völkerkunde, Berlin.

Bibliografische Information Der Deutschen Bibliothek:
Die Deutsche Bibliothek verzeichnet diese Publikation in der Deutschen
Nationalbibliografie; detaillierte bibliografische Daten sind im Internet
über http://dnb.ddb.de abrufbar.

Bibliographic information published by Die Deutsche Bibliothek:
Die Deutsche Bibliothek lists this publication in the Deutsche
Nationalbibliografie; detailed bibliographic data is available in the
Internet at http://dnb.ddb.de.

Printing and binding: Memminger MedienCentrum AG
Printed in Germany

www.harrassowitz.de/verlag
ISSN 1610-5354
ISBN 3-447-04600-7

To the memory of John and a wonderful journey.

VORWORT

Quellen und Forschungen zur Südsee ist eine Reihe, die Anstösse geben will, die wissenschaftliche Erforschung des Pazifik voranzubringen. Sie steht allen Arbeiten offen, die aus den Bereichen Geschichte und Geographie, Völkerkunde und Sprachwissenschaften, Religionswissenschaften, Biologie, Soziologie, Politikwissenschaften oder verwandter Gebiete stammen und die unsere Kenntnisse über den pazifischen Raum in beträchtlichem Maße erweitern oder korrigieren. "Südsee" wird hier relativ weit verstanden: Von Hawai'i und der Osterinsel im Osten bis zum ehemals niederländischen Teil der Insel Neuguinea und Palau im Westen. Im Norden bilden die Marianen die Grenze, im Süden sollen auch Australien und Neuseeland dazugehören.

Es ist ein besonderes Anliegen der Reihe, Forschungen in deutscher Sprache zu intensivieren und herausragenden Untersuchungen und Forschungsergebnissen eine Gelegenheit zur Veröffentlichung zu geben. Damit soll der wissenschaftliche Diskurs in deutscher Sprache über den pazifischen Raum verstärkt werden. Manuskripte, die in der sogenannten reformierten Rechtschreibung abgefasst worden sind, werden prinzipiell der Begutachtung nicht zugeführt. Bislang unveröffentlichte Arbeiten in Englisch können publiziert werden, sofern sie neben der selbstverständlich vorausgesetzten hohen wissenschaftlichen Qualität eine ausführliche deutsche Zusammenfassung enthalten. Vorschläge zur Veröffentlichung in der Reihe werden jederzeit entgegengenommen. Interessenten wenden sich an

Prof. Dr. Hermann Hiery
Lehrstuhl für Neueste Geschichte
Universität Bayreuth
95440 Bayreuth
e-mail:
Neueste.Geschichte@uni-bayreuth.de
Fax: 0921 5584 4181

Zur Einführung

Es ist kein Zufall, daß die *Reihe der Forschungen* mit einer Arbeit über das koloniale Gesundheitswesen in Neuguinea eröffnet wird. Untersuchungen zur Kolonialgeschichte, insbesondere deutschen Kolonialgeschichte der Südsee werden thematisch einen besonderen Schwerpunkt der Reihe bilden. Das koloniale Gesundheitswesen im Pazifik gehört zu den am wenigsten erforschten Bereichen der Kontaktgeschichte.

Margrit Davies ist eine geborene Schweizerin, die in Australien heimisch geworden ist. Die dort aufbewahrten deutschen Kolonialakten konnte sie deshalb auf dem Hintergrund einer umfassenden Kenntnis mitteleuropäisch-deutscher und pazifisch-insularer Vorstellungswelten und Verhaltensweisen auswerten und verarbeiten. Dr Peter Sack von der Australian National University in Canberra hat die Arbeit ursprünglich angeregt. Für ihre Veröffentlichung als Band 1 der *Quellen und Forschungen zur Südsee* wurde die Studie in wesentlichen Teilen erweitert und modifiziert.

Bayreuth, im Oktober 2002   Hermann Joseph Hiery

TABLE OF CONTENTS

Appendices

Tables

Maps

Illustrations

Conventions

There is no single English name to encompass the north-eastern part of mainland New Guinea, and I use the term 'Kaiser-Wilhelmsland'. This conforms with the situation during the German period, when Kaiser-Wilhelmsland and the Bismarck Archipelago formed two separate administrative units.

For place names of European settlements, I use German names and follow the *Deutsches Kolonial-Lexikon* for standardisation. For the islands of the Bismarck Archipelago I use present-day names, viz. New Britain = Neu-Pommern; New Ireland = Neu-Mecklenburg. German names used in the text and their modern equivalents are:

Eitape	Aitape
Friedrich-Wilhelmshafen	Madang
Herbertshöhe	Kokopo
Kaewieng	Kavieng
Stephansort	Bogadjim

Abbreviations

The first citations of archival collections and government publications are in full; abbreviations are used thereafter. They are as follows:

G/...	PNG Archives Government of Papua New Guinea, National Archives and Records. Records of the Imperial Government of German New Guinea.
AR	*German New Guinea: The Annual Reports,* translated and edited by P. Sack & D. Clark.
Draft AR	*German New Guinea: The Draft Annual Report for 1913-14,* translated and edited by P. Sack & D. Clark.
Amtsblatt	*Amtsblatt für das Schutzgebiet Neuguinea,* 1909-1914.
DKB	*Deutsches Kolonialblatt. Amtsblatt für die Schutzgebiete in Afrika und der Südsee.*
DKG	*Die Deutsche Kolonial-Gesetzgebung. Sammlung der auf die deutschen Schutzgebiete bezüglichen Gesetze,* 1893-1910.
MB	*Medizinal-Berichte über die Deutschen Schutzgebiete.* 1903/04-1912/13.
NKWL	*Nachrichten über Kaiser-Wilhelms-Land und den Bismarck-Archipel.*
RKA	Reichskolonialamt Records, Berlin. The designation RKA is used throughout for the records of the three authorities responsible for colonial matters—the Foreign Office up to 1890, the Colonial Department of the Foreign Office from 1890-1907, and the Colonial Office after May 1907.

Titles of the most frequently cited journals are abbreviated as follows:

ASTH	*Archiv für Schiffs- und Tropenhygiene*
DKZ	*Deutsche Kolonialzeitung*
JCH	*Journal of Contemporary History*
JPH	*Journal of Pacific History*
PNGMedJ	*Papua New Guinea Medical Journal*
VBG	*Verhandlungen der Berliner Gesellschaft für Anthropologie, Ethnologie und Urgeschichte*

ACKNOWLEDGEMENTS

I have had help and advice from many sources in the researching and writing of this study. My first thanks are due to Dr Peter Sack, who encouraged me to take up work on German New Guinea and generously gave me access to his collection of New Guinea materials.

Many other individuals have given me assistance in many different ways and I would like to make special mention of Dr Janitschke from the Robert-Koch-Institut in Berlin, Dr Stefan Wulf from the Bernhard-Nocht-Institut für Tropenmedizin in Hamburg, Professor Wolfgang U. Eckart from the Institut für Geschichte der Medizin, Universität Heidelberg, Dr Paul Weindling from the Wellcome Unit for the History of Medicine in Oxford, Frau Irmgard Duttge in Hamburg, Dr Hans-Michael Berenwenger in Stuttgart, and Dr Wigley in Sydney. Professor Donald Denoon and Dr Anthea Hyslop supervised me during the researching and writing of the thesis. They were always there when I needed to consult them and provided much valued critical guidance and support. I am indebted to all of them not only for the material they made freely available to me and the time they gave me, but also for their interest in my topic.

Irmgard Fox was unsparing in her encouragement and support during the revision of the thesis and also took the time to proof read the revised version; her help is greatly appreciated.

I also wish to express my appreciation for the willing help and friendly assistance I received from the staff of libraries and archives—the Australian Archives in Mitchell (ACT), the National Library of Australia, particularly the Newspaper/Microfilm Section, the Central Library of The University of Queensland, the library of the University of Erlangen, the Bundesarchiv, Abteilung Berlin, and the Senckenbergische Bibliothek in Frankfurt am Main.

The Australian National University granted me a full-time Master of Arts research scholarship and I am greatly indebted for this financial support. The thesis was completed at the end of 1992 and accepted in March 1993. It is published here with some revisions. The bibliography has been updated to include publications up to the beginning of 1998.

I am very pleased indeed that Professor Herman Hiery has accepted my study for publication in his new series *Quellen und Forschungen zur Südsee*. It is especially pleasing that he has chosen it as the first volume of the series. I am much indebted to him for his assistance in the final preparation of the manuscript.

Last, I am grateful to my family who took an unfailing interest in my work, and patiently and cheerfully put up with my stories of death and disease.

Although I have had much help from many sources, any mistakes in this work are my own.

INTRODUCTION

*We should not imagine that human skills can
arbitrarily transform a foreign region of the globe
into a Europe by cutting down its forests and
cultivating its soil, for all living creation is connected
and should be altered only with care.*[1]

This is a study of the evolution of public health policies in New Guinea
during the thirty years of German colonisation, from annexation in
1884 to the occupation by Australian troops in September 1914.
The Protectorate of the New Guinea Company was established with the grant
of an Imperial Charter to the company in 1885. It consisted of the north-eastern part of mainland New Guinea, which was called Kaiser-Wilhelmsland,
and the Bismarck Archipelago (the chain of islands to the north and north-
east). In 1886 the northern section of the Solomon Islands (the Shortland
Islands, Buka, Bougainville, Santa Isabel and Choiseul) were added. With the
transfer of power from the New Guinea Company to the Reich in 1899, the
territory became the Imperial Colony of German New Guinea. As part of the
Samoa Agreement in 1900 there was a border realignment in the northern
Solomons and only Buka and Bougainville remained German. These
Melanesian possessions became known as the "Old Protectorate" when the
so-called "Island Territory", comprising the Mariana and Caroline Islands
(purchased from Spain in 1898), was incorporated into the administration.
In 1906 the Marshall Islands, a German Protectorate which included
Nauru, was also incorporated into German New Guinea.

1   J.G. Herder, *Ideen zur Philosophie der Geschichte der Menschheit*, [c. 1784-1791], in vol. 9 of
     Herder's Werke, ed. H. Düntzer. (Berlin: G. Hempel, n.d.), 64. Except where otherwise
     indicated, translations are my own. I am grateful to Dr Margaret Stoljar for suggestions on
     translating Herder.

1

A comprehensive study of the wider territory called German New Guinea was not possible, and I concentrate my study on the Old Protectorate. A focus on Kaiser-Wilhelmsland and the Bismarck Archipelago seemed appropriate. This was a distinct administrative unit in German times, and its coastal regions—which was as far as German control extended—shared a common epidemiological climate.

New Guinea had experienced little contact with the outside world and was colonised relatively late. Not only was New Guinea isolated from the outside world: its communities were isolated from each other, which created a distinct epidemiological environment. Crowd infections, such as smallpox, measles, mumps, chickenpox, rubella and the common cold, could not exist in an isolated population as the survival of the virus depends on large populations, so that epidemics were most unusual. However, certain conditions— malaria, filariasis and yaws—were endemic, and it is highly likely that they were present from early times, with malaria a powerful factor in determining population size and distribution. Intestinal parasites probably came to New Guinea with the first invasion by humans or spread with gardening practices.[2] Endemic diseases, together with respiratory infections, bowel infections, skin infections and sepsis from trauma, were probably the main causes of sickness and death before colonisation.[3] The arrival of colonists was to change the epidemiological environment of New Guinea swiftly with the introduction of infectious diseases.

Health was possibly the last thing on the minds of colonial enthusiasts, but it soon became a central issue in the newly established settlement of Finschhafen in Kaiser-Wilhelmsland, when all newcomers—Germans and the small labour force brought along from the Dutch East Indies—became malaria infected. Malaria was the major threat to the survival of the settlement, but soon poor sanitary conditions and poor nutrition also began to have an effect as increasing numbers of labourers were brought in.

German immigrants did not rush to Kaiser-Wilhelmsland to take up land as the New Guinea Company had envisaged. Instead, the company decided to develop a plantation colony for which it took Java as the model. A large part of the labour force was imported from south-east Asia, mainly to grow tobacco, and from the Bismarck Archipelago and the Solomons for clearing

---

2   I. Maddocks, 'Communicable Disease in Papua and New Guinea', *PNGMedJ* 13.4 (1970): 120-4

3   I. Maddocks, 'Medicine and Colonialism', *The Australian and New Zealand Journal of Sociology* 11.3 (1975): 27

and other heavy infrastructure work. Illness and death claimed a heavy toll in the early years, and eventually the company had to abandon its attempts to create a second Java, concentrating instead on copra, the commodity which was the economic base for expatriate traders and planters in the Bismarck Archipelago. With erroneous assumptions, miscalculations and mismanagement, conflicting interests and also some plain bad luck, rule by a charter company was a failure and the colony could become viable only if the Reich assumed power, which it did in April 1899.

The transfer of power had implications for health services. One lesson from the company rule was that private enterprise was not suited to safeguard public health; company interests and doctors' responsibilities were often in conflict. Under imperial administration, doctors were employed as servants of the colonial state, responsible to the governor, and public health became a government responsibility.

During the years in which the New Guinea Company and the imperial government in Berlin were negotiating the return of the charter, progress was being made in medical research which was vital to the colony. The theory that miasmas—noxious vapours from putrescent organic matter which polluted the atmosphere— spontaneously generated malaria, had long been accepted, but already in 1880 the French bacteriologist Laveran had shown the malaria parasite in the blood. In 1894 Patrick Manson suggested that the mosquito was the vector for malaria, a hypothesis which Ronald Ross proved in 1897. Germany's most outstanding medical research scientist of the time, Professor Robert Koch, had been interested in malaria for many years, having worked on it in Calcutta and in Italy. The breakthrough by Ross encouraged him to continue his studies in the Dutch East Indies and in Germany's notorious "fever colony", New Guinea. In the six months he spent in Kaiser-Wilhelmsland he confirmed the work of Ross and other researchers and developed a method for the eradication of malaria based on quinine therapy and prophylaxis.

These were also the years in which 'tropical medicine' emerged, broadly defined as a medical speciality which focused on specific diseases occurring in tropical countries at the expense of other measures to ensure a general improvement in the health of all, and initially aimed at protecting Europeans from prevalent diseases in newly acquired tropical colonies.[4] What was forgotten when the colonial experiment began was that general

---

4   M. Worboys, 'The emergence of Tropical Medicine', in G. Lemaine et al, eds., *Perspectives on the Emergence of Scientific Disciplines* (The Hague/Paris: Mouton, 1976) 75-98

health improvements in Germany since early in the century had been achieved with a general rise in the standard of living, sanitary reforms and nutritional improvements.[5] In order to cope with these so-called "tropical diseases", German doctors were trained in the new medical speciality before leaving for a tropical colony.

There were many health problems to be addressed. They arose first of all because immigrants to Kaiser-Wilhelmsland had no immunity against malaria and local people were not immune against the crowd infections brought by the newcomers. Health problems were compounded by overcrowding, poor sanitation and poor nutrition.

Attention could not be limited to expatriates and immigrant labourers, for it was evident that introduced crowd infections were also spread to villages and hamlets. When the Reich assumed power, the colonial administration had to concern itself with long term planning for the development of the colony. The bulk of the population had to be included in these calculations for it was the source from which a growing labour force had to be drawn if the colony was to prosper; yet it seemed the source might run dry, for there were indications that the population was declining.

Against this background I shall explore a number of questions centering on public health. My study is a doctor-centred view, for much of my information comes from their reports and statistics. But there are certain problems with medical evidence.

Detailed morbidity records listed the number of patients and the type of diseases doctors treated, but I lack the medical expertise to interpret the diagnoses of the day, many of which, by doctors' own admission, were uncertain. However, I can look at broad categories of diseases from the perspective of public health and explore how doctors approached wider problems. Mortality records for Europeans are reasonably accurate as far as numbers are concerned, but cause of death has to be viewed with the same caution as morbidity records. Labour mortality records are particularly deficient for the New Guinea Company period, and for the later years the same reservations apply as for statistics on Europeans.

Up to the turn of the century the indigenous population was largely ignored, except for the smallpox crisis. When planners began to take the bulk of the population into consideration, it took years before doctors were able to go into villages to investigate the causes of the perceived population decline,

5   C. Huerkamp, *Der Aufstieg der Ärzte im 19. Jahrhundert. Vom gelehrten Stand zum professionellen Experten: Das Beispiel Preußens* (Göttingen: Vandenhoeck & Ruprecht, 1985) 135

assess health status, and devise ways of creating a demand for medical services.

Health questions relating to expatriates were widely discussed by all interested parties, but the discussion was one-sided when it came to labourers or the local population who, naturally, were not consulted. This leads to a curious situation in which we know the number of native hospitals Germans built and their dimensions; we know that doctors were in charge of hospitals, that German medical orderlies were responsible to the doctor, and that in turn coloured attendants were supervised by orderlies; but there is nothing to tell us how patients experienced hospital.

A number of aspects have been left out. One omission is a discussion of the medical work of missions who devoted much effort to giving help to New Guineans. However, missions are considered whenever they had an influence on shaping government attitudes and policies.

The financial aspects of health administration have been omitted also. For the New Guinea Company period, no financial records survive. Occasional comments on the company's health expenditure by contemporary writers were guesswork. The household budgets for the Imperial Government are complex and need a separate study. I have therefore made no systematic analysis of health finances, but simply mention some details.

Census lists proved another blind alley. The two categories 'adults' and 'children' were by the administration's own assessment unreliable, as distinction between them was a subjective judgement of the surveyor. For some districts, the census figures were the result of several counts, and in others they were estimates. Altogether, there was not enough information—despite long lists—to draw up an age related population profile or establish with certainty whether the contemporary view of a population decline was correct.

The first chapter examines doctors working in German New Guinea, their values and attitudes, their professional organisation, and some of the non-medical problems they encountered. In the second chapter I deal with some of the health problems encountered by Europeans in New Guinea and measures taken to protect them from disease. I also discuss the expectations expatriates developed and their prior claims on the health care system. The third chapter examines the health of the labour force. Starting with a short discussion of labour mortality rates, I go on to explore medical influences and financial interests that determined health policies for the labour force. In the fourth chapter I discuss effects of colonisation on the health of the native population, the crucial status health gained for the economic survival of the colony, and policies devised to halt a population decline. In conclusion I discuss some of the issues that arise from an overview of the three groups of health services consumers.

The evidence is clear that Germany's handling of health was in line with the practice of tropical medicine. This focused on specific diseases at the expense of general health. However, by 1914 it had become obvious that wider measures had to be taken to ensure better health for all people under German control. The economic viability of the colony depended not only on the health and well-being of expatriates and labourers, but on a healthy population. Treating diseases alone was insufficient to improve public health.

1

COLONISATION AND THE
MEDICAL PROFESSION

Not even the European diligence of civilized
colonies can always avert the effects of the climate in
other parts of the world.[1]

This chapter focuses on doctors[2] and the "fully furnished world they brought with them"[3] to German New Guinea. Their values, assumptions and beliefs, and their work, were shaped as deeply as anybody else's by the culture and time in which they lived. Underpinning the work of doctors were medical and sociological theories current in Germany during its colonial period, and for this reason they bear examination.

An important factor that engendered the proliferation of these theories was the increasing prestige, influence and power of doctors in Germany, with major advances in scientific research in the 1870s and 1880s: the discovery of asepsis and antisepsis, of bacteria as the cause of a specific disease, and of diagnostic innovations. In Germany doctors grew confident and powerful enough

---

1   Herder, *Ideen zur Philosophie der Geschichte der Menschheit* 64
2   The term 'doctor' is generally used as a translation for *Arzt*. The title *Doktor* applies to someone with a doctorate in any discipline. The English term 'physician' excludes surgeons and therefore has misleading connotations. In this I follow Paul Weindling's usage of the term in his *Health, Race and German Politics between National Unification and Nazism, 1870-1945* (Cambridge: CUP, 1989)
3   To quote G. Dening, *Islands and Beaches: Discourse on a Silent Land, Marquesas 1774-1880* (Melbourne: MUP, 1966) 224

by the 1880s to launch an aggressive campaign against quackery and gain a monopoly on health care. With it they waged a campaign to extend the scope of scientific medicine not only into health but also the social spheres of life.[4]

One manifestation of medical theorising was the emergence of 'tropical medicine', the integration of doctors into this new medical speciality, and with it the direction taken by doctors in the colonies. Another theory that gained increasing currency was that of racial hygiene. It also found an echo in the way doctors perceived their task of intervening in the health of New Guineans.

These theories, and the scientific, economic and social developments that gave rise to them, were not limited to Germany. In the second half of the nineteenth century similar processes were under way in other European states. This is not to suggest that developments or effects of increasing medical influence on the health of the people were identical in each country; but this is not the place for a comparative analysis of these developments. What was similar was the rising prestige of the medical profession, and its influence and power throughout western Europe. In his detailed study of the rise of the medical profession in Prussia in the nineteenth century, Huerkamp makes the point that while the "professionalisation" of doctors occurred throughout western Europe, Great Britain and the United States, as a result of medical training in state controlled institutions there was a significant difference in Prussia and other German states, in that the medical profession was much more closely tied to the state than in Britain and the United States.[5] This point is confirmed in the colonial context. Eugenic movements also became active throughout Western countries. Evolving within different traditions, developments took diverse paths, especially after 1918.[6] Similarly tropical medicine as a speciality was not simply a German phenomenon, but has to be viewed within the broader context of European imperial expansion into tropical colonies, notably by Britain and the Netherlands.[7]

4   Weindling, *Health, Race and German Politics* 16-21
5   Huerkamp, *Der Aufstieg der Ärzte*, 15-16. For the rise of the medical profession in England see, for instance, F. B. Smith, *The People's Health 1830-1910* (Canberra: ANU Press, 1979) especially 362-82
6   It has been suggested that Anglo-American eugenics was largely private and supported by philanthropy, but German race hygiene evolved within a statist medical tradition. For this and the development of eugenics in non-English speaking countries, see M.B. Adams, ed., *The Wellborn Science: Eugenics in Germany, France, Brazil, and Russia* (Oxford, Oxford UP, 1990) 4
7   For the development of tropical medicine in Britain see M. Worboys, 'The Emergence of Tropical Medicine: a Study in the Establishment of a Scientific Speciality', in G. Lemaine et al, eds. *Perspectives on the Emergence of Scientific Disciplines*, (The Hague: Mouton & Co., 1976) 75-98. For the similar development in the Dutch context, see G.M. van Heteren

In the first part of this chapter I analyse medical theories dominant when Germany began its colonial experiments. The first is the theory of acclimatisation; the second relates to the discovery of microorganisms as pathogens. The evolution of tropical medicine from these theories as a scientific speciality and its institutionalisation in Germany are then discussed.

This is followed by a brief discussion of the theory of racial hygiene in Germany. Although this theory was developed on the basis of social and economic conditions in Wilhelmine Germany, it reverberated also in German New Guinea, and a perceived decline of the indigenous population was, at least in part, explained in eugenic terms. It also became a factor influencing the development of colonial health policies.

In the second part I turn to German New Guinea and look at some of the doctors and their attitudes to the indigenous population. The employment of doctors is then discussed by focusing on some of the doctors and the problems they encountered, and their influence, or lack of it, on health policies.

MEDICAL AND SOCIOLOGICAL THEORIES

When Germany annexed its colonies, it was accepted that climatic influences determined directly and indirectly the health of people. According to this theory, physical well-being was optimal in the climatic conditions in which a person was born. On the home ground physical disposition, determined by racial or national characteristics, was in complete harmony with all external influences which affected an individual. Nevertheless, experience had taught that certain people had the capacity to adjust to foreign climates so that they could live there without damage to physical health. Such adjustment was seemingly based on certain permanent changes in the body's metabolism— a gradual modification of biological processes, the so-called "acclimatisation". In this sense "colonisation" meant the complete adjustment of people from a certain race or nationality to a foreign climate, so much so that they could

---

et al, eds., *Dutch Medicine in the Malay Archipelago, 1816-1941* (Amsterdam: Atlanta, 1989) especially the chapter by van Heteren, 'The course in tropical medicine at Amsterdam: 'a case of monopolisation'?' 35-56; and de Knecht-van Eekelen's chapter 'The interaction of western and tropical medicine' 57-72. For a discussion of the possibility that colonial powers differed in their approaches to tropical medicine, see Worboys' chapter 'British colonial medicine and tropical imperialism: a comparative perspective', 153-168

increase through procreation and settle permanently. It followed that acclimatisation was easier and more complete the less the differences between native climate and new surroundings, irrespective of race, so that 'the tropics' were the very opposite of German climatic conditions, and therefore the most dangerous to health and the most difficult to which to adjust.[8]

The question of acclimatisation of Germans in the new colonies was first taken up at a meeting of the *Berliner Gesellschaft für Anthropologie, Ethnologie und Urgeschichte* [Berlin Society for Anthropology, Ethnology and Prehistory] in May 1885 by its president, Rudolf Virchow. He was the leading German pathologist, a prominent left-liberal politician and anthropologist. Much to his surprise *the* fundamental question in the acquisition of colonies had not been mentioned at all in German colonial literature, neither by colonial propagandists nor by economists, although British, Dutch, and French experience had shown that any colonial activity was impossible unless there was some understanding of the effect of the climate on the human body, in particular the capacity of Europeans to adapt to a tropical climate.[9]

Virchow subscribed to the current theories of miasmatic emanations as the cause of malaria, but pointed out that, although high ambient temperatures and malaria were often found together, there were areas of high temperature where there was little or no malaria, and cool regions which were malarial. The difficulty for Europeans was to find malaria-free places for settlement. As for the German colonies, the medical geographer Hirsch, in his epidemiological study[10] published in 1881, had established that the coast of New Guinea was highly malarial, but that the islands of the Bismarck Archipelago were less so, and the Polynesian islands malaria-free. Virchow doubted the accuracy of Hirsch's information, but sounded a strong warning that all indications pointed to a very virulent malaria in New Guinea, raising serious doubts about its suitability for European settlement. He also warned against the erroneous belief that a person could get accustomed to malaria, for it was characteristic of malaria that attacks increased in gravity leading eventually to malaria cachexia.

---

8   A. Hirsch, 'Acclimatisation und Colonisation', *Verhandlungen der Berliner Gesellschaft für Anthropologie, Ethnologie und Urgeschichte,* (VBG) (meeting 27 February, 1886), 18 (1886): 156-57
9   R. Virchow, 'Acclimatisation.' VBG (meeting 16 May, 1885), 17 (1885): 202
10 A. Hirsch, *Handbuch der historisch-geographischen Pathologie,* (Stuttgart, 1881). The second edition of the book was translated into English by C. Creighton, and published in 3 volumes under the title *Handbook of Geographical and Historical Pathology,* by the New Sydenham Society, London, 1883-1886.

He was not at all sanguine about the possibility of eradicating malaria, pointing to the difficulties with attempts outside Rome and suggested that an eradication program in a tropical country with primeval forests would be much more difficult than in the relatively accessible Roman countryside.[11] His pessimism, though based on wrong theories, proved well founded.

Virchow took up European acclimatisation again later in 1885, when he addressed a much wider audience, the *Vereinigung Deutscher Naturforscher und Aerzte* [Society of German Naturalists and Doctors] (VDNA). This society, similar to the British Association for the Advancement of Science, provided a national forum for scientific debates. It was one of a number of scientific societies in which professional and amateur scientists and other members of the middle-class shared their interests and within which scientific programs were canvassed.[12] Together with other liberal anthropologists Virchow opposed the acquisition of colonies. From an anthropological point of view, colonies threatened the survival of many cultures; from a political point of view colonies were costly, risky and useless.[13] However, much as he disagreed with the political goals, he could see the possibilities for scientific work in colonies and the role that science could play there:

> This is not the place to discuss whether we should become a colonial power; we will become one, and natural and medical scientists will not be able to passively stand by a process decided upon by the government. The government as well as the nation are fully justified in demanding answers from science for a whole range of questions which will be decisive about the ways and directions to be taken in the formation of the new colonies. It will be absolutely necessary that science provides the basis for the new communities overseas.[14]

Virchow claimed a fundamental place for science in the new colonial enterprise. It was to guide the establishment, management and development of colonies; it was the key to successful colonisation because it promised to provide answers to colonial problems.

Another health warning was sounded at the next annual meeting of the VDNA, this time by Hirsch. Experience of other colonial powers had shown that even under the most favourable conditions a European "suffers the loss

---

11   Virchow 208-210
12   Weindling 29
13   Weindling 57
14   Quoted in E. Cohn, 'Zur Geschichte der deutschen Tropenhygiene', *DKZ* 17 (1900): 53

of his strength, physical and intellectual capacity to work are reduced ... and in all tropical countries a European will suffer illness and early death if he occupies himself with the cultivation of the soil." Northern Europeans were unable to acclimatise in tropical or subtropical countries. Agricultural work by an immigrant in such countries led to illness and early death. If Germans wanted to emigrate they should choose a relatively mild climate, free of malaria; but people should be warned against "all utopian hankering after emigration."[15]

These warnings, delivered to people from the educated middle-class, did not dampen colonial enthusiasm. The mere fact that these questions were raised by known anti-colonialists would have discounted them. In any case, there was also the promise that science would produce solutions. The fast pace of bacteriological discoveries suggested that such promises were grounded on a sound scientific basis.

Virchow only slowly conceded ground on miasmatic theories. However, he did not waver from his contention that epidemics were not solely bacteriological, but also social in their causes, and that there was a close connection between medical science, economic interests and political ideology.[16] These views on public health might well have given food for thought to colonial doctors and administrators. Virchow himself did not relate his theories to the colonial context; but, as his biographer pointed out, he preserved the concept of sociological epidemiology, even when the overwhelming concern with bacteriology appeared to make the search for any other causative factor unnecessary.[17]

From today's vantage point it seems a great pity that Virchow's theories on epidemics fell into abeyance by the time German administrations had to deal with epidemics in the colonies. From the beginnings of colonisation different strategies might have been developed to deal with public health crises.

When Virchow and Hirsch raised these questions Robert Koch was also at work. His theories had greater influence on the development of health policies. His reputation was well and truly established through his work in isolating the anthrax bacillus in 1876, his subsequent discoveries of the tuber-

---

15   Hirsch 164-166
16   R.J. Evans, *Death in Hamburg: Society and Politics in the Cholera Years 1830-1910* (Oxford: Clarendon Press, 1987) 274-5
17   Virchow formulated his views on public health early in his career, following his trip to Upper Silesia in 1848 to investigate a typhus epidemic, and further elaborated them following a cholera epidemic in 1848-49. E.H. Ackerknecht, *Rudolf Virchow, Doctor, Statesman, Anthropologist.* (Madison: University of Wisconsin Press, 1953) 126-128

culosis bacillus in 1882, and the cholera bacillus in 1884. In 1880 he had been provided with a laboratory at the Imperial Health Office (*Reichsgesundheitsamt*) in Berlin, where he made his most celebrated discoveries. He had also been appointed to the new chair of hygiene at the University of Berlin in 1885. In 1891 the government provided him with his own research institute, the Institute for Infectious Diseases in Berlin.[18] In a political sense, the timing of Koch's discoveries was crucial. The scramble for Africa had begun; Germany had imperial ambitions to compete with other European powers. Nations, engaged in a race to annex territories in the name of civilisation, were also engaged in furious competition to conquer disease in the name of science. Koch's discoveries enhanced Germany's reputation for outstanding scientific work. With his record Koch was the most influential adviser in colonial health matters and had close associations with the government, becoming a government adviser (*Regierungsrat*) with the Imperial Health Office in 1880. Before the Institute for Tropical Diseases was established in Hamburg, Koch trained a number of students in principles and techniques of bacteriology in preparation for their medical work in the colonies in his Berlin institute.[19]

The advantages of Koch's bacteriological theory over Virchow's were simplicity and elegance. The way to combat and eradicate disease was to find and identify the pathogen, then attack and destroy it. Virchow argued for an interplay of a number of factors. Involved were not only pathological causes, but also social conditions, economic interests, and political will. None of these lent itself readily to scientific analysis, or to a simple solution, nor to the imposition of centralised measures; planners had to be cognisant of local variations of social, economic and political circumstances. The fact that Koch's theories prevailed in the Imperial Health Office had consequences also in the development of colonial health policies for many years.

18   G. Olpp, *Hervorragende Tropenärzte in Wort und Bild* (Munich: Otto Gmelin, 1932) 206-7

19   Among those were doctors going to German New Guinea: Hintze arrived in Friedrich-Wilhelmshafen 23 April 1901; Dempwolff, who was sent by Koch to continue the investigative work on malaria, arrived 17 October 1901; Jacobs arrived July 1900 in Stephansort; Ollwig, who accompanied Koch on the malaria expedition; Seibert, who took up work in Herbertshöhe in 1905 also worked at the institute for some months.

Tropical Medicine as a Medical Speciality

Tropical Medicine was one of the medical specialities to emerge late in the nineteenth century.[20] The concept of tropical medicine was propagated, professionalised and popularised in a systematic manner. In the early colonial period, the term 'tropical hygiene' encompassed health and ill-health of Europeans living in the tropics. When colonial administrators began to concern themselves with the health of the indigenous population, the term came to include all peoples in tropical colonies. The terms 'tropical diseases' and 'tropical medicine' came into use gradually, probably influenced by their use in Britain, initially in the *Journal of Tropical Medicine*, first published in 1898.[21]

When the question of European acclimatisation was brought to the attention of the *Deutsche Kolonialgesellschaft* [German Colonial Society],[22] it was not only as a warning of the dangers to the health of Europeans, but also as a way to enlist support for scientific research. As the scientific interests of the VDNA and the practical interests of the Colonial Society coincided, it was natural that the two bodies should co-operate on the question of European acclimatisation. From its inception, doctors were members of the Colonial Society. From a total of at least 144 doctors and teachers at university medical schools in 1889, their number increased steadily and by 1903 some 1500, that is five percent of German doctors, were members.[23] Whatever the ideological reasons for this support, colonies also provided work for many doctors and medical scientists—no mean consideration since

20 Huerkamp notes that a number of medical specialities began to emerge from the 1880s on, all based in the large cities: ophthalmology, ear nose throat specialists, skin and venereal diseases, nerve specialists, women's diseases, surgeons, children's specialists. Treatment of internal diseases remained the domain of the general practitioner. Huerkamp 178 ff

21 H. Jusatz, 'Wandlungen der Tropenmedizin am Ende des 19. Jahrhunderts', in G. Mann & R. Winau, eds., *Medizin, Naturwissenschaft, Technik und das Zweite Kaiserreich*, 227-38 (Göttingen: Vandenhoeck & Ruprecht, 1977)

22 The German Colonial Society was founded in 1887, an amalgam of the *Deutscher Kolonial-verein* [German Colonial Association] and the *Gesellschaft für Deutsche Kolonisation* [Society for German Colonisation]. The former was an association in which individual and corporate interests from industry, commerce, banking, politics and science were represented. The association advocated and promoted German colonial expansion. The Society for German Colonisation was founded by Carl Peters, adventurer and explorer in Africa, and supporters with similar objectives. The foundation membership of the Colonial Society was nearly 15000, and grew to around 43000 by 1914. It proved to be one of the large and powerful pressure groups of the Wilhelmine era. R.V. Pierard, 'The German Colonial Society' in A.J. Knoll & L.H. Gann, *Germans in the Tropics*, 19-37 (New York: Greenwood Press, 1987)

23 S. Parlow, 'Ueber einige kolonialistische und annexionistische Aspekte bei deutschen Ärzten von 1884 bis zum Ende des 1. Weltkrieges', *Wissenschaftliche Zeitung der Universität Rostock* 40 (1966): 537

there was an overproduction of doctors in Germany by 1900 and their number had all but doubled since 1876.[24]

In the 1880s scientific research relating to health in the tropics focused on
investigating specific local climatic conditions, on the basis of which counter-
measures could be taken. Detailed meteorological measurements and details
of types and incidence of disease and mortality were recorded and collated,
seeking correlations between climate and diseases. Physiological functioning
of people of differing races was measured and compared. This pattern was so
firmly established that, even when miasmatic theories were discredited, discus-
sions on the acclimatisation of Europeans continued unabated, and meteorological data were included in annual medical reports for several years.

When the 1889 VDNA meeting approved a questionnaire, compiled by a
number of doctors and scientists, to gather this fundamental information, it
was sponsored by the Colonial Society and was sent out to doctors in tropical and subtropical countries. The results of the survey, published by the
Colonial Society, were discussed at the annual assembly of the VDNA in
1891, but only thirty-three of the two thousand questionnaires had been
returned, insufficient to support any conclusions. A lack of statistical material
on the tropics made a response to the questionnaire nearly impossible. A
revised questionnaire had similar unsatisfactory results, leading the 1894 meeting of the VDNA to the conclusion that fundamental questions of the survival
of Europeans in the tropics could not be established by schematised questions.
Scientific laboratories were needed where underlying physiological laws could
be observed and studied, where German scientists could carry out research
similar to that at British and Dutch institutes.[25]

Unfavourable publicity surrounding the acclimatisation of Germans in the
tropics, no doubt reinforced by adverse reports from the colonies through private channels, together with the propaganda by the Colonial Society and the
VDNA, created a suitable climate for submitting a proposal to the Reichstag
for the establishment of institutes for tropical hygiene. The Reichstag
response was positive and the Imperial Health Office was directed to take the
matter in hand.[26]

It took another four years before the Reichstag allocated funds for the
establishment of an institute for tropical hygiene.[27] During that time the original

---

24 The number of doctors rose from 13,738 to 27,374. Weindling 17
25 *DKZ* 10 (1893): 51. Below, 'Bericht 66. Versammlung Deutscher Naturforscher und
    Aerzte', *DKZ* 11 (1894): 145-6
26 Below, 'Bericht 67. Versammlung Deutscher Naturforscher und Aerzte', *DKZ* 12 (1895): 324
27 *DKZ* 16 (1899): 106

proposal was modified in a significant way on the recommendation of Koch: instead of a research institute in each tropical colony, one Reichs-institution was to be established under the administration of the Colonial Department.[28] Located in Berlin, close to the centre of Koch's work, the aim of the institute was the health and welfare of Europeans; it was to be set up as a research and teaching institute where doctors could prepare for work in the tropics and where Germans returning from the colonies could be restored to health.[29]

However, before details were completed, a counter-proposal came from Hamburg. The chief medical officer of Hamburg and the doctor in charge of the medical supervision of the harbour, Dr Nocht, proposed that the work of the Seamen's Hospital should be reorganised, so that only patients suffering from tropical diseases would be treated there. They would be "the material" for clinical observation at a new institute, designed specifically for research on tropical diseases. The Senate of the City of Hamburg had adopted the proposal and made funds available. Following lengthy negotiations between the Reich and the Hamburg Senate, an Institute for Ships and Tropical Diseases was established in Hamburg, where it opened on 1 October 1900.[30] The City of Hamburg agreed to fund the institute with an initial outlay of 253,000 Mark in addition to a first budget for 1901 of 104,000 Mark; and the Colonial Department paid a subsidy of 10,000 Mark.[31] This subsidy increased over the years[32] and entitled the Colonial Department to sponsor doctors to attend training courses in tropical medicine in Hamburg.[33] The arrangement between the City of Hamburg and the Reich apparently did not give rise to any recriminations because of Hamburg's disproportionate financial contributions—Nocht knew how to

28 The Colonial Department was at that time a branch of the Foreign Office. The Colonial Office was established in 1907 with Bernhard Dernburg as Colonial Secretary, following a reorganisation of the colonial administration. Present at the meeting which adopted the new proposal were the Colonial Society, represented by von Arenberg; the Colonial Department of the Foreign Office (von Buchka, director); Prof. Robert Koch as director of the Institute for Infectious Diseases; Prof. Sachau, a member of the *Kolonialrat* [Colonial Couincil]; Hpt. von Laurens (seconded from Colonial Troops to Colonial Department); Dr Nocht, in charge of the Harbour Doctor's Office [*Hafenarzt*] and Chief Medical Officer of the Seamen's Hospital in Hamburg; Dr Kohlstock, *Referent* in the medical branch of the Colonial Office and a close colleague of Koch's; Dr Schön, Imperial Health Office.

29 *DKZ* 16 (1899): 106-7

30 *ASTH* 4 (1900): 11ff; *DKB* 11 (1900): 649

31 20 Mark were the equivalent of £1 sterling

32 J. W. Spidle, *The German Colonial Civil Service: Organisation, Selection and Training*, diss., Stanford University (Ann Arbor: University Microfilm, 1972) 294

33 *DKZ* 18(1901): 173

exploit Hamburg's civic pride.[34] The work of the institute grew rapidly; by 1905 it had to be enlarged, only to be found too small a few years later. Following a decision in 1910, the City of Hamburg spent 2,320,000 Mark on a new complex which was opened at the beginning of 1914.[35] The annual budget for the institute had increased to 246,000 Mark.[36]

In the early years of the institute there was frequent reference to British research in tropical medicine and the schools for tropical medicine in Britain. It appears that there was much more government involvement in Germany, in the form of representation both by the Colonial Office and the Imperial Health Office, than there was in England[37] where, according to Professor Fülleborn from the Hamburg institute, "the munificence of the English mercantile interests" provided funds for employing a large number of researchers and financing tropical expeditions. In contrast, the Hamburg institute was very much involved in teaching activities and the lack of researchers meant that a lot of research material could not be fully used.[38] As only first class research would guarantee a world-wide reputation, Fülleborn was keen to enlarge the research function of the institute at the expense of teaching. However, the level of teaching was maintained. Between 1901 and 1913, 790 doctors underwent training at the Hamburg institute. Of those over forty percent were directly in the employ of the Colonial Office, the Colonial Troops[39] and the Navy.[40] The large number of private doctors suggests that many hoped to make tropical medicine a career. In addition to the two courses per year for doctors, courses were introduced for medical orderlies and nurses from the German Women's Association for Nursing in the Colonies.[41] Despite the emphasis on training the Hamburg institute quickly established the highest reputation; the London *Spectator* in 1914 called it "the greatest [institution] of its kind in the world"[42], and it has maintained a high reputation to this day.

34 Spidle 295
35 Nocht, *ASTH* 18 (1914) Beiheft 5: 20
36 *Deutsches Kolonial-Lexikon* II: 100–101
37 See Worboys 75-98
38 F. Fülleborn, 'Reisebericht über einen Besuch der tropenmedizinischen Schule in England', *ASTH* 8 (1904): 298-99
39 The Colonial Troops (*Schutztruppen*) were independent from the German military and naval forces, but part of the overall German armed forces, under the command of the Secretary for Colonies, who in turn was responsible to the Chancellor and ultimately to the Emperor. There were no Colonial Troops in German New Guinea. *Deutsches Kolonial-Lexikon* III: 321-4
40 Archival file from the Bernhard-Nocht-Institut für Tropenmedizin in Hamburg (formerly the Institut für Schiffs- und Tropenkrankheiten)
41 *Deutsches Kolonial-Lexikon* II: 100–101
42 Cited in Spidle 289

The 1901 course program for doctors was based on the need to diagnose and treat tropical diseases, and to carry out research on such diseases. Doctors were instructed in the techniques of preparing and examining blood samples, and the examination of *anopheles* and *culex* mosquitoes. Instruction on malaria was extensive, covering etiology and diagnosis, morphology and development of malaria parasites, symptoms and progress of diseases, treatment of malaria and blackwater fever, and animal malaria. Similarly intestinal diseases (such as dysentery), intestinal parasites, typhus, cholera, diphtheria, and plague were covered. Students were also taught to examine and assess drinking water. Quarantine and ships' hygiene was another topic. The program was not entirely laboratory based as there were two weekly clinical visits, depending on the cases hospitalised.

By 1904 the course program was lengthened to six weeks to include animal diseases—but only one weekly clinical visit—and by 1908 the course was extended to eleven weeks. Malaria remained the main topic. Two days were allocated to 'tropical hygiene'; new also were morphology and biology of spirochaetes, yaws, buboes, tropical phagedaenism, and verruca peruviana. Animal diseases were given eight working days. Again, there was only one weekly clinical visit.[43] It seems that the program emphasised research rather than clinical work. However, in the public health area it was obviously important that a doctor be able to identify cholera or plague bacilli and carry out water testing. Staff members from the institute also undertook thirteen research expeditions to various parts of the globe, two of them to the Pacific.[44]

It took fifteen years from the time Germany became a colonial power to the establishment of an institute of tropical medicine. It took less time for another manifestation of its institutionalisation—the publication in 1897 of the journal *Archiv für Schiffs- und Tropenhygiene*. The impetus came from the VDNA, an initiative welcomed by the Colonial Department, the Imperial Health Office, and the German Colonial Society.[45] Carl Mense, a doctor who had worked in the Congo and then took up private practice in Hamburg, was its editor from 1897 to 1916.[46] The journal, in its early years

43   Archival file from the Bernhard-Nocht-Institut für Tropenmedizin in Hamburg
44   The first was in 1908/09 under the leadership of Prof. Fülleborn, the second in 1910/11 by Prowacek and Leber to combat eye diseases in the Island Territory of New Guinea and Samoa. Nocht, 'Das neue Institut für Schiffs- und Tropenkrankheiten', *ASTH* 18 (1914) Beiheft 5: 23
45   C. Mense, Die deutsche Tropenmedizin vor 25 Jahren und später. *ASTH* 25 (1921): 3
46   Olpp 280

bi-monthly, grew very quickly; in 1901 it appeared monthly, and from 1907 on a number of supplements (*Beihefte*) were also published, most of which contained lengthy original articles. In the first year of publication, fifteen major articles appeared, at least seven of them from doctors practising in German colonies and the Dutch East Indies. The main topics were malaria, beriberi, and leprosy. The journal settled down quite quickly to what was to become its basic format: each issue contained two or more original articles, a section entitled 'pathology and therapy', which provided a forum for discussion on many aspects of tropical diseases, and a section for book reviews and brief notes about matters from other colonial powers. Malaria continued to be a major topic, but beriberi, dysentery, leprosy, yellow fever, plague, skin diseases, and later on helminthic diseases were all discussed. There were also occasional articles on public health such as water supplies and eradication of mosquitoes.[47]

In addition to training at the same institution and subscribing to the same specialist journal, doctors formed the *Deutsche Tropenmedizinische Gesellschaft* [German Society for Tropical Medicine] in 1907.[48] When invitations were sent out for the first plenary meeting in April 1908, there were sixty-seven members, of whom twenty-nine were doctors in the Colonial Troops or in the Navy; ten worked at the Hamburg Institute for Tropical Diseases and three at the Berlin Institute for Infectious Diseases; of the two government medical officers who were members one had worked in New Guinea.[49] By the time the meeting was held, membership had increased to one hundred and seven. At the same time as the founding of the German Society for Tropical Medicine, an International Society for Tropical Medicine was founded during the Hygiene Congress in Berlin, in September 1907. Its founders believed that there was much common ground among European colonial powers and that a free exchange of research among these nations would benefit all.[50]

The professional circle is completed when it is considered that all quarter-

---

47 For example, by G. Giemsa, 'Trinkwasserverhältnisse und Trinkwasseruntersuchungen in den Kolonien', *ASTH* 7(1903): 447-55; 'Beitrag zur Frage der Stechmückenbekämpfung', *ASTH* 15(1911): 533-5; 'Das Mückensprayverfahren im Dienste der Bekämpfung der Malaria und anderer durch Stechmücken übertragbarer Krankheiten', *ASTH* 17(1913): 181-90

48 P. Kuhn, 'Fortschritte der Tropenhygiene', *DKZ* 24(1907): 410

49 Dr Seibert from February 1905- May 1907. Membership list in *ASTH* 12 (1908): 180-182

50 Sander, 'Bericht 75. Versammlung Deutscher Naturforscher und Aerzte', *DKZ* 25 (1908): 292

ly and annual reports from doctors working in the colonies to the Colonial Office were sent on "for information" to the Institute for Ships' and Tropical Diseases in Hamburg and the Institute for Infectious Diseases in Berlin. This ensured feedback on clinical results of research, but was probably more useful as general information on the state of health in the colonies, or as a guide in the selection of projects.

Awareness by the lay public of the concepts of tropical diseases and tropical medicine was also fostered. At the International Hygiene Exhibition in Dresden in 1911, visited by millions of people, it was given wide publicity through large displays. The Hamburg institute displayed much of its teaching material. The public was enlightened about malaria through large models and panels depicting the malaria cycle. Photographs of the Trypanosoma Expedition could be contemplated, as could pictures of all types of tropical skin diseases. There was a particularly rich display of tropical intestinal parasites—nematodes and trematodes in macroscopic and microscopic forms— and the many tropical diseases affecting animals. Of great interest was the collection of tropical snakes, fish, spiders, and scorpions, together with sera developed against their bites or stings. There were pictures and models of tropical houses, water supply systems, tropical clothing and nursing care in the tropics. There was also a display of native staple foods, together with analyses of their nutritional values. Undoubtedly the highlight of the tropical section was the New Guinea house on stilts with a life-size group of native people in front of it, gathering sago, palm oil and sorghum.[51]

A particular image was created for popular consumption to show life in the tropics and the role of scientific research in paving the way to eliminating the dangers and horrors of tropical diseases. The public was familiarised with the 'otherness' of tropical diseases and with tropical medicine. The exhibition clearly demonstrated the close link between colonies, "where Germans fought for health and life"[52] and medicine.

Racial Hygiene and the Colonial Economy

From the 1880s the concept *Rassenhygiene* (racial hygiene) developed out of theories of Social Darwinism. The first stage of this development lasted until 1914.[53] Some notions of racial hygiene found an echo also in the considera-

---

51 M. Mayer, 'Tropenhygiene und Tropenkrankheiten auf der Internationalen Hygiene-Ausstellung zu Dresden', *ASTH* 15 (1911): 785-88
52 C. Mense, 'Die deutsche Tropenmedizin vor 25 Jahren und später', *ASTH* 25 (1921): 2
53 Weindling 9

tion of colonial health policies. Its relevance to New Guinea is discussed in a later chapter, but a broad outline of racial hygiene theories and their colonial context is appropriate at this point.

The development of racial hygiene theories in Germany needs to be seen in the context of Germany's rapid industrial development, a surge in population growth and urban expansion, and the resulting social, economic and political problems. The biological and medical ideologies that prevailed in the educated middle class (*Bildungsbürgertum*), the scramble for power and social influence by the medical profession, and the interaction of interest groups with state authorities all played a part in the development and adoption of theories of racial hygiene.[54] The concern here is with the early history of racial hygiene, which at that time was distinct from the ideology of a superior Aryan race.

Racial hygiene seemed to offer solutions to the pressing problems of the time. Analogies were drawn between biological units and social organisation, and biological observations were used to justify social roles. Pioneering work in experimental cytology and embryology in the 1880s showed heredity as a hidden factor which shaped social life, and a debate ensued about biological heredity. Although infectious diseases such as cholera and typhus were declining, "racial poisons" such as alcoholism, tuberculosis and venereal disease were perceived as damaging the nation's hereditary stock. High rates of venereal disease were found especially in large cities, and they were seen to lead to either infertile marriage or diseased offspring. The notion of a hereditary disposition to tuberculosis persisted despite Koch's proof that it was a contagious disease; alcoholism was seen to result in decreased fertility, weakened progeny and high rates of infant mortality. Other chronic or inherited diseases, such as short-sightedness, diabetes, and neurological complaints—even dental caries—indicated a decline in the quality of the population.

In the 1870s and 1880s the view had been that Germany was overpopulated and as a result many emigrated; prevention of population loss became one of the themes of colonial propagandists. By the turn of the century this view was reversed; the demand for labour was increasing and fears of underpopulation were expressed. Because of rapidly increasing life expectancy and high fertility from 1870 on the population had been growing at a fast rate. From around 1900 there was a marked decline in the birth rate, typically manifested first in the

---

54 The German term *Rassenhygiene* encompassed both the notion of improving hereditary qualities of a population and notions about measures designed to increase the size of the population. The English term 'eugenics' corresponds to the first notion. See S. Weiss, 'The Race Hygiene Movement in Germany', *Osiris* 2nd series, 3 (1987) : 193-198

industrial urban population. A population decline was perceived as another threat to German society, a sign of degeneration, as morally and physically pathological, with serious implications for the military and economic power of the nation. Medical intervention at childbirth and infant care were advocated as ways of reducing maternal and infant mortality and infant morbidity.[55] Diverse as the factors were that gave rise to racial hygiene theories, the underlying view was that "population was a resource amenable to 'rational management'". Eugenicists equated fitness with productivity and achievement, and degeneration with asocial behaviour and the inability to contribute to society.[56]

The racial hygiene movement was formalised as a pressure group with the founding of the *Gesellschaft für Rassenhygiene* [Racial Hygiene Society] in 1905. The membership was middle-class, almost exclusively professional, open to a select group with high mental and physical qualities, some forty per cent coming from the medical or medically related professions.[57] The anthropologist Richard Thurnwald, an expert on New Guinea, was a founding member, as was Dr Külz, who was appointed Chief Medical Officer for German New Guinea in 1913.[58] As members of the professional middle class, they shared views on social problems; doctors in particular perceived their role as safeguarding the health of the nation. With the rise of scientific medicine, the medical profession gained not only in social esteem but also indirectly in political importance. It also gained control of the conditions of medical practice and was able to dictate what was good health.[59]

The notions of overpopulation and population decline were also reflected in colonial debates. Part of the rhetoric for Germany's need for colonies had centred on the 'loss' that Germany ostensibly suffered because of the large number of emigrants. German territory had to be found overseas for these emigrants so that they would remain part of the German nation: there would be no population 'loss'. It was also accepted wisdom that there were native populations available in tropical countries, both as a labour force for German

---

55   This outline is based on Weindling 173-5, 189-90, 241-246
56   Weiss 195, 203
57   Weindling 141-2
58   Other members of the society with New Guinea connections were the anthropologist Rudolf Pöch, who spent 12 months in Kaiser-Wilhelmsland and the Bismarck Archipelago in 1904 to 1905 for anthropological, ethnographic and medical studies; the geographer Karl Sapper, who studied New Ireland and its people in 1908; also Dr Siebert who visited German New Guinea for two months and advised the government on health conditions in northern New Ireland. I am grateful to Dr Weindling, who made available to me a list of the members of the Racial Hygiene Society.
59   Weindling 20-21

settlers and as prospective consumers for German manufactured goods. If some colonies were seen as having an unlimited supply of native populations, this view changed when it became obvious that epidemics introduced by Europeans caused high death rates. Chronic diseases were seen to affect a large number of native people, and they reduced the capacity to work; the number of children in a family was observed as being generally smaller than in Germany. By the time voices were heard about a population decline in Germany, the same state of affairs was perceived in the colonies. As in Germany, so in the colonies, low fecundity was seen as a sign of degeneration. The decline and destruction of whole populations was considered to be the inability of an inferior race to adapt to a higher culture, or to withstand the impact of a higher race. Although a high native population density had never been attributed to German New Guinea, the same general pattern was perceived. If anything, the situation there was seen to be worse because of the relatively small base population.

Besides eugenic notions on population decline, I would suggest that another factor came into operation in the colonies. By the turn of the century, scientific research promised that malaria eradication was close. Among colonial interests this raised the prospect of permanent settlement in malarial regions and with it the opening up of more land for plantations to meet the ever increasing demand in Germany for raw materials. More plantations created the need for a larger labour force at the very time when population decline was taken as a fact. A decreasing population, or one unable to work because of ill health, would threaten the prospects of plantation colonies as much as malaria had done.

In order to solve "the population problem" and on the basis that economic progress, population growth and public health were closely linked, from around 1905 onwards a number of doctors practising in the African colonies began to put forward proposals for a comprehensive public health system for the indigenous populations of the colonies. Initially the debate took place in medical circles, in particular the second meeting of the German Society for Tropical Medicine in 1909.[60] From there the issue was

---

60   To cite the main proponents: (1) Külz, 'Der hygienische Einfluss der weissen Rasse auf die schwarze Rasse in Togo' [The hygienic influence of the white race on the black race in Togo] *Archiv für Rassen- und Gesellschaftsbiologie* 2.4 (1905); (2) H. Ziemann, 'Wie erobern wir Afrika für die weisse und farbige Rasse?' [How do we conquer Africa for white and coloured races?] *ASTH* 11 (1907) Beiheft 5; (3) H. Ziemann, 'Ueber die Errichtung von Tropeninstituten und die Gestaltung des ärztlichen Dienstes' [The establishment of tropical institutes and the organisation of medical services] *ASTH* 13 (1909) Beiheft 6: 46–54; (4) C. Schilling, 'Der ärztliche Dienst in den deutschen Schutzgebieten' [Medical services in the German colonies]. *ASTH* 13 (1909) Beiheft 6: 32–45

taken up in wider colonial circles, at the Third Colonial Congress in 1910.[61] To complement the debate Dr Külz, then a senior government medical officer in Cameroon, also discussed the question in an article published in the *Deutsches Kolonialblatt*. He further elaborated on the topic in the medical and the eugenic press.[62] As this debate also affected the views of doctors in German New Guinea, its main points are considered briefly.

At the Colonial Congress and in Külz's article, the question of public health of the indigenous population was discussed in essentially economic terms. The main speaker at the Colonial Congress, Dr Schilling, emphasised that without an indigenous labour force well acclimatised to working in a hot climate, tropical colonies were "dead capital", nothing other than "a heavy burden" on the colonising power. The latter found itself needing the indigenous population "unconditionally", if it did not want to see its colonising efforts "wasted fruitlessly".[63] Külz argued his case in similar terms. "If I were asked", he began, "what the main goal of all colonial work in our tropical colonies was, I would reply that it is to open them up economically ... and to create new economic values." He went on to say:

> Given it is an economic axiom [in Germany] that the most valuable capital of the state is its population, this applies to an even greater extent to the indigenous populations of a tropical colony. Any successful development depends above all on them; they are the producers of exports and the consumers of imports; they are the labour force for European enterprises as well as the producers of their own economic output.[64]

As in Germany, so in its colonies, the population was seen as a resource of the state. Like any other resource it had to be managed to ensure its full productive capacity, to "lift the level of fitness" by promoting optimum conditions.

---

61 C. Schilling, 'Welche Bedeutung haben die neuen Fortschritte der Tropenhygiene für unsere Kolonien?' [What do new advances in tropical hygiene mean for our colonies?] *Verhandlungen des Deutschen Kolonialkongresses 1910*: 162-185. L. Külz, 'Wesen und Ziele der Eingeborenenhygiene in den deutschen Kolonien', [Nature and objective of native hygiene in the German colonies] *Verhandlungen des Deutschen Kolonialkongresses 1910*: 342-56

62 L. Külz, 'Die Volkshygiene für Eingeborene und ihre Beziehung zur Kolonialwirthschaft und Kolonialverwaltung' [Public health for natives and its relationship to the colonial economy and administration], *DKB* 21 (1910): 12-21. 'Grundzüge der kolonialen Eingeborenenhygiene', [Outlines of native public health in the colonies], *ASTH* 15 (1911), Beiheft 8. 'Beitrag zum Bevölkerungsproblem unserer tropischen Kolonien', [The population problem in our tropical colonies] *Archiv für Rassen- und Gesellschaftsbiologie* 7.5 (1910)

63 Schilling, 163

64 Külz (1910) 12

As in Germany, doctors claimed the right to intervene; they were the "appointed guardians of native peoples".[65] Külz used arguments similar to those of the eugenic movement to justify medical intervention and control.

Schilling and Külz agreed that colonisation had adverse effects on the health and social fabric of indigenous populations. Traffic among native tribes and populations had increased considerably since colonisation, as pacification opened the way for closer inter-tribal relations. Many natives worked in transport enterprises, carrying not only goods but also diseases. Enormous numbers of labourers from many disparate regions were gathered in one place to work on plantations or on road construction; others were part of expeditionary forces. Despite precautions and medical treatment, labourers were seriously affected by changes in climate, nutrition and accommodation, and by unfamiliar work. These changes in lifestyle predisposed them to infections which spread readily in cramped living conditions. Despite obvious health problems in the labour force, lay people were still under the misapprehension that natives adjusted well and quickly to new surroundings. There were also indirect deleterious effects of recruitment in villages. The absence of thousands of young people often had the unfortunate consequence that food supplies were affected. Yet another effect was the reduction in births due to the absence of males in the marriageable age group.[66] Külz spoke of his observations in African colonies, but many of the problems listed also prevailed in German New Guinea.[67]

Külz knew only too well that a colonial doctor faced difficulties in trying to come to grips with health issues. The main problem was that he had to fulfil the dual, often conflicting, roles of general practitioner and public health officer. A doctor provided immediate treatment for an individual, usually seen by the administration and lay people as the main function of a doctor. "Handing out an effective medication, or a bandage, or carrying out a successful operation are well understood [by the native] and are to his or her liking, and will chain that person closer to us than raising taxes or road construction." In this sense medical work was "playing colonial politics" and medicine was a means to an end, a sure way of fostering trust in Europeans. However, treatment of individual patients paled in comparison with the work

---

65   ibid.
66   ibid. 15–16
67   In the African context, Külz pointed to the severe problems with alcohol. As the sale of alcohol to natives in German New Guinea was effectively prohibited from the time of annexation and alcohol did not become a public health issue during the German administration, this point need not detain us here.

of a public health officer, even if, as a general practitioner, he successfully treated a thousand people a year who could then resume work. This had little impact on the economy, if at the same time whole villages died out because of epidemics.

The fundamental objectives of public health, Külz noted, were the same in the colonies as in Germany, although specific difficulties were encountered with public health measures in the colonies. One was that they were opposed by colonists if they appeared detrimental to their immediate economic goals. Another was the great gap between the objectives of public health and what was feasible with the resources allocated for the purpose. Nevertheless it was essential that public health was part of an administration's program as each new district was opened up. Creating healthy conditions for labourers and troops on stations, followed by clean water and sanitary facilities for villages had to be the first concern of any administration and no doctor was needed for the implementation of these public works. As for combating disease, Külz's view was that, rather than piecemeal work on all fronts, it was better to target some specific problems. For a start smallpox should be eradicated in all colonies; dysentery, leprosy and (in Africa) sleeping sickness should be attacked urgently but attention to problems like skin diseases should be postponed until more urgent work had been carried out.[68] Overall, Külz advocated a two-pronged approach, a combination of sanitary measures and mass campaigns against infectious diseases rather than an attack on diseases alone as had been the practice in the first twenty or so years of the colonial experiment. Essentially he proposed that measures similar to those which had improved general health in Germany during the nineteenth century should be implemented in the colonies.

Implicit in Külz's program was the need to educate Europeans both in the colonies and at home. Colonists had to have a better understanding of the cost-benefit aspect of good labour conditions, to realise that investment in improvements was cost-efficient. At home, parliamentarians and other influential bodies had to apply pressure, so that the Reichstag was favourably disposed to allocating money for public health in the colonies. In the context of New Guinea the master plan of Külz is discussed in the last chapter.

68   Külz ibid. 13, 19-20

DOCTORS IN GERMAN NEW GUINEA

The published and unpublished writings of doctors who worked in German New Guinea reveal their attitudes towards the indigenous population, the influences they brought to bear, how their work changed and how they handled it.

During the early part of the New Guinea Company operations, doctors were not occupied fully with medical work and spent time on ethnography. Few people were in their care and they were limited in what they could treat. The main problem was malaria: there was no cure for it, and in mild cases neither Europeans nor labourers sought a doctor's help, but looked after themselves. When hospitals were built, they were simple in construction and lacked equipment for complicated surgery, although operations under full anaesthetic were not unknown. Even when the number of labourers increased, a doctor's work was monotonous, with malaria, dysentery, influenza, beriberi, and tropical sores part of the everyday routine. Quarantine duty was not onerous as the number of ships was small. As the number of Europeans and labourers increased, so did the work load, and after the turn of the century there were changes in the doctors' work. In theory they were to become part of a scientific research network; in practice all they could do was report clinical observations and results. But, as hospitals became better equipped, more complicated surgery could be carried out; medical examination and care of labourers became more time-consuming as numbers increased; shipping traffic increased considerably and with it the health inspection of ships; medical reports to the Colonial Office became more complicated; visits had to be paid to Europeans at considerable distances from a doctor's residence; and increasingly attention shifted to the health of the indigenous population. There was no longer time for ethnographic studies such as were carried out in the days of Schellong and Hagen. These had become the task of the numerous research expeditions that descended on German New Guinea.[69] Most of the doctors who worked in German New Guinea published articles in medical journals concerning clinical cases. Of equal interest here are their non-medical publications and by way of example those of Drs Schellong, Dempwolff and Hagen are briefly examined to show their main interests and concerns.

---

69   For example, the Hamburg South Seas Expedition 1908-1910; scientific expeditions to the Bismarck-Archipelago by Sapper and Friederici in 1908; German Naval Expedition 1907-1909; Richard Neuhauss spent 18 months in Kaiser-Wilhelmsland in 1909-1910. Although the focus of their research varied, all included ethnological research.

Otto Schellong

The first German doctor in New Guinea, Otto Schellong, published extensively and, on his return from Kaiser-Wilhelmsland, quickly became known as an authority on tropical medicine and New Guinea through articles which he wrote both for the colonial press and for medical journals. Popular articles dealt with the acclimatisation of Europeans, with advice on accommodation, food, clothing, life style, and coping with malaria. Articles in medical journals discussed malaria in its clinical aspects, both as he experienced it in the 1880s and his views after 1900. He also published a number of articles in leading ethnographic journals and a book on the Yabim language. His memoirs, based on his diary, were published in 1934 when he was seventy-six years old, nearly fifty years after his stay in Kaiser-Wilhelmsland from January 1886 to April 1888.

Schellong was optimistic when he set out for New Guinea: "I don't need to make out more than one report a month, I have plenty of medications for two years ... and as far as my work is concerned, I will fulfill my duties and follow my conscience, as any good doctor does."[70] Reality was not quite as straight forward: one medical problem came up with regular monotony—malaria. Apart from dispensing quinine, he could not do much other than speculate on possible causes and take regular climatic measurements in the hope that statistical material would eventually provide clues. He was well aware that he was powerless to do much about malaria, and he left New Guinea in great disappointment, feeling that he had not been effective as a doctor and healer.[71]

As medical work did not keep him fully occupied, he spent quite some time on ethnography for which he had an abiding interest. With the help of his medical orderly he made plaster casts of twenty-four Yabim people from the surrounding villages (in the area of Finschhafen), and more in other areas.[72] His contract with the New Guinea Company did not allow him to sell artefacts or any other ethnographic material to museums or collectors. Such items were, so to speak, collected in company time, and they belonged to the New Guinea Company.[73] Schellong also took detailed somatic mea-

---

70   O. Schellong, *Alte Dokumente aus der Südsee: Zur Gründung einer Kolonie* (Königsberg, 1934) 32

71   O. Schellong, 'Die Neu-Guinea Malaria einst und jetzt', ASTH 5 (1901): 303

72   O. Schellong, 'Beiträge zur Anthropologie der Papuas', *Zeitschrift für Ethnologie* 23 (1891): 158

73   The New Guinea Company sold 40 of these, made from people from neighbouring villages from Finschhafen, from Tami-Island, New Ireland and New Britain, as well as samples

surements of thirty-seven Yabim, a survey that was done with the help of standard ethnographic charts designed by Virchow.[74]

His articles on the Yabim people and his memoirs give a distinct impression that he was sympathetic, that he liked them as a people, and many of them as individuals. They impressed him first of all by their intelligence: "They are a highly intelligent people. We should not believe that we have people from the stone age here who are a long way from any culture. Their language is very rich ... they have an excellent musical ear ... and much can be said about their manual and artistic skills".[75] He also admired their crafty negotiations for trade goods. Yet a solid wall of incomprehension separated him from the Yabim, exemplified in the story of Ssanguan, a village elder, well known to Schellong. When he heard that Ssanguan was dying, Schellong went to see him and found him "courageously awaiting his death". His family and friends were gathered around the dying man, but no attempt was made to save him from death.[76] Schellong's suggestion that he be given some fortifying food was ignored. Incomprehension was apparently mutual: the relatives could not understand his suggestion, his wanting to take action; he could not understand their lack of action—it was as if they were looking at different events. Yet what could Schellong have done? If it was pneumonia, he would have been as helpless as the people who had gathered around, "a quiet, grave and dignified group";[77] his suggestion was more in the nature of a reflex action that was not likely to change the outcome.

As for personal cleanliness of the natives, Schellong speculated that dirt, mainly caused by smoke drifting over the sleepers inside the huts at night, created protection against mosquito bites; it was "a protective layer, not a dirt layer". The cleanliness of the villages impressed him, be they villages in the Finschhafen area such as Suam, or along the Bumi river where a small group of houses and a native plantation "struck very pleasantly in their cleanliness".[78] Perhaps they compared favourably with the peasant villages of his native West Prussia.

    of hair and a number of skulls to the Berlin Museum of Anthropology for 500 Mark in 1889 (*VBG* meeting 18.5.1889).

74 Schellong, 'Beiträge' 158-230

75 O. Schellong, 'Mitteilungen über die Papuas (Jabim) der Gegend des Finschhafens', *Zeitschrift für Ethnologie* 37 (1905): 602-18 and *Alte Dokumente* 54

76 From Schellong's description, Ssanguan was dying from bronchiopneumonia: fever and racking cough, exhaustion, falling into semi-conscious state out of which another coughing fit would shake him up.

77 O. Schellong, 'Ueber Familienleben und Gebräuche der Papuas', *Zeitschrift für Ethnologie* 20 (1888): 20

78 Schellong *Alte Dokumente* 42-45, 64

His attitude towards the Yabim is conveyed in his 1905 article, where he noted how quickly they adopted and used items from the new civilisation which suited their purposes and made work easier than their traditional tools. When he arrived some six weeks after the first contingent of settlers, the local people had already put aside their stone axes and tools made from shells and bones and were using iron axes to fell trees. Within a year the Yabim no longer accepted cheap trade axes but demanded proper axes. Similarly with glass and matches: these were adopted quickly and were soon found at considerable distances from European settlements.[79] Schellong accepted the changes as a matter of course; he did not express regret that they were happening so fast that Europeans did not have time to study the population in depth in their 'original' state. The Yabim were not simply an object of European study; they remained individuals with individual differences. In this regard Schellong was in the mould of Virchow and other liberal anthropologists who saw their role as one of recording differences among the human population, differences which exemplified the immense potential for human variation.[80]

It could be expected that Schellong would write extensively about medical aspects in the life of the Yabim. He attended to natives in surrounding villages from very early on, but treated mainly sores and ulcers. He was mystified—as were many after him—that people should think they did him a service when they let him bandage their sores.[81] He noted that sorcery was seen as the cause of illness and misfortunes. Often an influential man in a neighbouring village had cast a spell which could be countered with another spell. He also noted "a complete lack of any medication".[82] He realised there were dimensions in the life of the native population that neither he nor other Europeans understood and saw great need to investigate these in a joint effort by missionaries, ethnographers and anthropologists, if there was ever to be any cultural understanding.[83]

This brings us to his article 'The German in Kaiser-Wilhelmsland and his attitude to the natives', in which he discussed the question of natives as a labour force and set out a 'native development plan'. The basis for this plan was the view typical of a colonist that Europeans needed cheap labour for their plan-

79   Schellong, 'Mitteilungen' 603-4
80   See Weindling 55, for details on the views of liberal anthropologists
81   Schellong, *Alte Dokumente* 63
82   Schellong, 'Ueber Familienleben' 19-20
83   O. Schellong, 'Der Deutsche in Kaiser-Wilhelmsland in seiner Stellungnahme zum Landeseingeborenen', *DKZ* 6 (1889): 69-86

tations and that such labour was available from "the lower coloured races".

Schellong argued that the precondition for a successful relationship between a European and a coloured labourer was that the latter did not see the former "merely as his master but essentially as his benevolent friend and caring guardian". As the "coloured children of nature" needed to learn about the puzzling world and ways of Europeans, they were badly in need of such a guardian who would direct them so as to avoid vice and excess that was part of white civilisation. Schellong took it for granted that indigenous peoples had to work for colonists, although he regarded it as essential that Europeans behaved in a humane manner and took measures to ensure decent conditions for labourers. In the Pacific colonies there should be a concerted effort by planters, missions, ethnographers and anthropologists to teach natives to work. However, he was in no doubt that the manner of recruiting labour raised some awkward questions. He strongly rejected coercion, but was not prepared to discuss just how much pressure could or should be put on natives to enlist for work. He noted that experience had shown that training could not be carried out on the natives' home ground, that they needed to be away from their home environment to get used to work. Clearly accepting the need to remove prospective labourers from that environment, he nevertheless saw it as all the more essential that labourers were accommodated properly and well catered for. He suggested that single men should be housed in native style houses for about fifty people and married couples should be allocated small houses of their own. While people had to get used to punctuality and learn to live and work by the clock, work should be appropriate to an individual's physical strength and varied, not restricted to one type of plantation work only. A school for tradesmen should be established, for their innate craft skills would make it easy to teach them to use European tools and train them as carpenters, smiths, or in other trades. Women should be trained to keep their houses clean, to sew, do laundry and practise other domestic skills, and Schellong assumed that European women would like to take on the job of teaching native women.[84]

In this 1898 article Schellong's attitude towards natives was rather paternalistic: the colonist was a fatherly figure, friendly but strict, the natives children who were allocated their place and in need of teaching how to fit into a society ruled by colonists. His plan, while reasonable to some planters, may well have dismayed others as being too liberal and generous, but all would have agreed with him that the fundamental objective was to make natives useful to

84   ibid.

Europeans and that the type of training he suggested would be a step in that direction. It is striking that Schellong did not see natives as individuals, unlike in the case of the Yabim that he had got to know. 'Natives' had become an anonymous aggregate of people, there to be taken into the service of the colonists.

In his 1889 article Schellong was addressing colonists and in particular the New Guinea Company, quite a different group from readers of ethnographic or medical journals and hence quite a different tone of language. Although he was critical of the ways recruitment was handled—he had seen enough of recruitment and labour conditions to know that there were serious problems—neither did he diverge from the view that natives had to be integrated into a colonial economy, nor did he see it as other than inevitable that the higher European civilisation would dominate; the question was how to find the most humane way to achieve the goal. If he was trying to direct colonists to ways which might avoid the excesses that he had observed, he was certainly treading carefully and he was anxious not to upset his former employer, the New Guinea Company.

Otto Dempwolff

Another doctor to take up the labour question was Otto Dempwolff, who worked in Friedrich-Wilhelmshafen from March 1895 to February 1897. In 'The education of Papuans as labourers', he offered a solution to the problem of inducing the indigenous population to join the plantation labour force.[85] He distinguished between the Tamul people living around Astrolabe Bay, and the Melanesians from the Bismarck Archipelago, saying that "the Tamul only accepts from the European civilisation those items of which he can make good use within his traditional economy, whereas the far more congenial Melanesian can be influenced much more readily, one can appeal to his sense of honour, and he shows at least some zeal to adjust to the wishes of the white man."[86] As applied psychology seemed to be helpful in getting Melanesians to work, Dempwolff set out a psychological approach to setting up such a system.

In Dempwolff's view colonists had to blame themselves for the lack of

85 Dempwolff, 'Die Erziehung der Papuas zu Arbeitern', *Koloniales Jahrbuch* 11 (1898): 1-14. (A less literal translation, but one more in the spirit of the article would be 'Teaching New Guineans to work'.) The nomenclature for the indigenous population was not fixed at the time. The term "Papua" was used by some to refer to the people of Kaiser-Wilhelmsland, by others to refer to all New Guineans (as Dempwolff did in his article); the term "Melanesian" usually referred to people from the Bismarck Archipelago, but was later also used to refer to all New Guineans.

86 ibid. 6

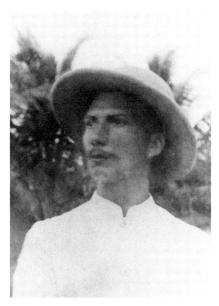

Dr Otto Dempwolff
in Friedrich-Wilhelmshafen, 1895

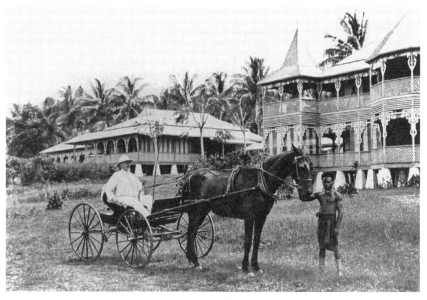

Dr Wilhelm Wendland in Herbertshöhe, 1906

co-operation from the Tamul; they had shown themselves to be very vulnerable as they needed any surplus food that could be produced locally. The newcomers also wanted artefacts and were prepared to pay ever increasing prices for them. Inflation had set in: in Stephansort the price for a coconut had risen to two sticks of tobacco, whereas in Friedrich-Wilhelmshafen it cost only half a stick; a number of axes were now demanded in exchange for woven shields from Karkar Island. The situation was paradoxical: Europeans should be in control, but instead they were dependent on the local population who exploited the situation when what they should do was work in plantations, as they were perfectly acclimatised and suffered far less from malaria and other diseases than labourers from the Bismarck Archipelago.

Dempwolff suggested that the way out of this predicament was for colonists to become as independent as possible from the natives, particularly in the supply of fresh food, which meant that plantation managements needed to grow fresh food for labourers on the plantations.[87] The trade in artefacts should be controlled, either by monopoly or by price fixing. By adopting such measures, natives would have to take up day labour in order to earn the cash necessary for their needs. The Tamul had shown that natives had developed weaknesses: they had become fond of rice; they preferred stick tobacco to their home-grown tobacco; and they preferred red lead paint for decorating their bodies in place of red ochre, all items for which they would be prepared to work. The next step should be to promote competition and ambition among individuals by training some as team supervisors for contract work. In Dempwolff's view, the introduction of his plan would lead to a system that had been used successfully by the Dutch for a long time, namely the execution of European rule through effective and responsible intermediaries who organised natives in small polities and provided compulsory labour in exchange for protection and administration. He argued that there was no need for Europeans to justify such a course of action; endowed with higher intelligence, they had the right to usurp control and to induce lower races to use their physical strength to open up and put to use the treasures of the tropical wilderness.[88]

As the two examples demonstrate, doctors had no hesitation in involving themselves in issues other than medical ones from the earliest days of colonisation. There is no way to measure the influence of articles on 'the native question' by men with a medical background. But doctors were held in high

87 This, as will be shown in the third chapter, was sound advice, but for other reasons.
88 ibid. 10-13

regard in Germany and their opinions and advice were taken seriously; articles of this nature were likely to propagate and confirm widely held evolutionary theories and ideas about 'the lower races' and the intellectual superiority of the white race.

Bernhard Hagen

Another doctor who published his memoirs was Bernhard Hagen[89] in 1899, with observations mainly on the Astrolabe Bay area and its people, the Bogadjim. He arrived in Stephansort in November 1893 to work for the Astrolabe Company (a subsidiary of the New Guinea Company) and left fourteen months later in January 1895 because of ill health. His thirteen years' experience as a doctor on tobacco plantations in Sumatra seemed to make him a perfect choice to work among plantation labourers in Astrolabe Bay, most of whom were Javanese and Chinese. He spoke their language and was familiar with their customs; hence he would be much more useful than a doctor with no plantation experience.[90] It was assumed by the company that health problems on tobacco plantations in Sumatra were identical with those in the Astrolabe Bay, and Hagen in turn arrived with certain assumptions about tropical colonies.

He arrived in New Guinea convinced that it was only a matter of overcoming the initial years of hardship for New Guinea to become a flourishing colony. He also expected that "each tropical colony has to be fertilised with human bodies before its fruit can be gathered, and Kaiser-Wilhelmsland is not the worst one in this respect, as some of the tropical diseases which are the main killers such as beriberi, cholera, and bubonic plague are not endemic, and malaria is not extremely virulent in character."[91] Hagen was in no doubt that sacrifices had to be made to the greater glory of the tropical colony, and that New Guinea was demanding its share of propitiatory gifts. From a medical aspect it is interesting that he categorised beriberi, cholera, bubonic plague, and malaria as 'tropical diseases'. To understand the spuriousness of conflating these diseases in this category, it needs to be remembered that malaria was still endemic in parts of Germany[92] and a severe cholera epidemic in Hamburg,

---

89 B. Hagen, *Unter den Papua's: Beobachtungen und Studien über Land und Leute, Thier- und Pflanzenwelt in Kaiser-Wilhelmsland* (Wiesbaden: Kreidel Verlag, 1899)

90 *NKWL* 1893: 34

91 Hagen 15

92 O. Schellong, 'Das Tropenklima und sein Einfluss auf das Leben', *Koloniales Jahrbuch* 5 (1892): 65. Also Mühlens, 'Malariabekämpfung in Wilhelmshaven und Umgebung', *ASTH* 13 (1909): 166-73, for malaria epidemics in 1902, 1907 and 1908 in northwest Germany of which the German public heard and knew nothing. L.J. Bruce-Chwatt

which had claimed nearly nine thousand lives in 1892, was still vivid in German memory.[93] On the other hand, at the time Hagen was writing his book, Robert Koch was visiting New Guinea on a malaria expedition, giving credence to the belief that malaria was a specifically tropical disease.

Hagen arrived during the smallpox epidemic in the region of Astrolabe Bay, so he had immediate contact with natives from surrounding villages. His reaction to "the bearded chaps with their wild, coarse cannibal faces" was one of disdain and ridicule. They observed smallpox vaccination "with a terrified rolling of the eyes" and responded to the small scratch from the blade "with a frightened jerk of the whole body, miserable wincing, and tears". He had no difficulty accepting that the vaccination procedure was seen by natives "as an act of sorcery, something utterly incomprehensible", but he left the reader in no doubt that he despised what he regarded as craven behaviour.[94]

The main body of Hagen's book is an ethnographic study of the Bogadjim people. Like Schellong, he took many somatic measurements; he also collected clay pots in the village of Uija, in the hinterland of Astrolabe Bay, to compare them with those collected by Finsch from Tami Island. The Bogadjim proved to be one of the oldest forms of human society, "a primitive people that was kept for us by a benevolent fate as an irreplaceable example from which we can form a vivid picture of the intellectual life of our own ancestors thousands and thousands of years ago."[95] The local people were an object which allowed Hagen to study different stages of a general evolution of mankind.

Communication

Hagen and Dempwolff both wrote about medical practices of natives, mostly based on information obtained from missionaries. It is not surprising that doctors relied on missionaries who had much closer contact with the indigenous population. Language posed a great problem; doctors were not there long enough to elicit much direct information on such complex subjects as ill health and disease.

Communication with patients was also difficult. The usual language

devotes one chapter to the history of malaria in Germany in his monograph *The Rise and Fall of Malaria in Europe* (Oxford: OUP, 1980) 82-88.

93   see Evans, *Death in Hamburg*, for an analysis for cholera epidemics in Hamburg from 1830-1910.
94   Hagen 41
95   ibid. 278

between Germans and natives was Pidgin, or "Coastal Malay" on stations such as Stephansort, while the labour force was predominantly Asian. Until such time as new arrivals—doctors or labourers—learnt a common language, medical practice closely resembled that of a veterinary surgeon. In the early days, when doctors' contracts were cut short for a number of reasons, few doctors were there long enough to learn to communicate properly with their patients, although diagnosis depended on a patient being able to respond to a doctor's questions. In the early years doctors felt in any case ill equipped to deal with the conditions they confronted because of assumptions that the pathology of people born in the tropics differed from that of Europeans; they were unsure of their diagnosis, as unsure as they were of the therapy that they prescribed in the hope that it would do no harm.[96] In many cases a diagnosis was possible only with an autopsy, and many were carried out over the years.

Working in isolation, doctors took avidly to writing and publishing articles in the *Archiv für Schiffs- und Tropenhygiene*. In the early days this was one way to share their professional experience. With the advent of the Hamburg Institute for Tropical Disease, and the training provided there, doctors grew increasingly confident that they could cope with the medical conditions confronting them in the colonies.

Organisation of Medical Services

Doctors worked in the colonies right from their establishment by Germany. In the African colonies where troops were stationed, military doctors were appointed, and they were responsible also for the civilian population. In German New Guinea doctors were employed by the company and, on transfer of authority to the Reich, the government appointed doctors under the similar terms as government medical officers in Germany. A list of doctors who worked in New Guinea and brief biographical notes are in Appendices I and II.

Under their conditions of contract, doctors had to take care of the health of all Europeans employed by the company, their families, and all company labourers. As well as the overall administration of hospitals, doctors were responsible for implementing and supervising quarantine measures (*Sanitätspolizei*). Monthly reports had to be submitted to the directors in Berlin on medical activities and the state of health in general, via the local company administration.

---

96   O. Dempwolff, Aerztliche Erfahrungen in New Guinea, *ASTH* (1898): 280; 291-2

When agreement was reached for the handing over of the administration of German New Guinea from the New Guinea Company to the Reich, to be effective as from 1 April 1899, the question of medical staffing and hospitals remained open and was subject to a separate agreement between the Reich and the company. In the meantime, the two company doctors, one in Friedrich-Wilhelmshafen and one in Herbertshöhe, continued working as company employees, and patients were treated in hospitals maintained by the company, with the government paying the New Guinea Company a daily fee for patients in government employ.[97]

The first government medical officer appointed was Wendland, who took up work in Herbertshöhe in November 1901. Hoffmann, the first government medical officer in Friedrich-Wilhelmshafen, began work in August 1902. For the remainder of the German period, medical staffing remained at one doctor in Kaiser-Wilhelmsland, but in the Bismarck Archipelago there was a gradual increase in the number of doctors. Early in 1904 a doctor was based permanently at Kaewieng; in 1905 a second doctor was appointed for the Herbertshöhe/Rabaul district. In Namatanai a permanent doctor took up work in 1911, and in Kieta in 1913. With the transfer of government to Rabaul, medical services were centred there, with two permanent doctors by 1913, in addition to a chief medical officer who was to take up his position in 1914.

With the appointment of government medical officers, an agreement was reached between the New Guinea Company and the government whereby the company paid an annual lump sum for services rendered by doctors. In Kaiser-Wilhelmsland this amount was the largest part of the doctor's salary, 7100 M; the government contribution to his salary was 2500 M. In the Bismarck Archipelago the amount paid by the company started off at 2500 M and increased to 4500 M by 1912; the same amount was paid by the Forsayth Company to the government after Rudolf Wahlen took over the company in 1911. Smaller plantation owners and the missions used the services of the government medical officer for which they had a private agreement with the doctor.

Salaries for doctors in the colonies ranged from 8200 M to 13900 M including overseas allowances, plus free accommodation. The guaranteed minimum income for a colonial doctor was usually 9600 M per annum. A posting to German New Guinea was for a 3-year period after which time a doctor was entitled to 4 months (excluding travelling time) home leave if

97   RKA 5729: 5-7; 17-20

he renewed his colonial posting. Doctors were directly responsible to the governor or his deputy. The medical service in New Guinea was reorganised in 1913/14 with the appointment of a Chief Medical Officer to head medical services, a new section within the administration. The Chief Medical Officer was to be responsible to the governor for all medical services including its staff. In practice the new set-up did not come into operation.[98]

The provision of health services was a considerable recurring cost. With the move of the seat of government to Rabaul in 1910, Governor Hahl proposed that government medical services be closed down in Herbertshöhe and that a private doctor be encouraged to set up practice. Contracts with well established private firms, able to provide medical services for their labour force without government subsidy, would guarantee a doctor a minimum income.[99] As was to be expected, there was local resistance from settlers and missions, fearful of higher medical costs.[100] The Centre Party in the Reichstag supported the settlers.[101] The Colonial Office also had reservations: at a time when the need for improved health services for the native population was recognised, it was important that the government was able to direct doctors to intervene and provide health care for the indigenous population.[102] The Colonial Office had little faith in the philanthropy of doctors and assumed they would not treat villagers free of charge as was government policy, if they were prepared to treat them at all. The result was that the medical services at Herbertshöhe were maintained at existing level—a doctor, a nurse, a medical orderly, a European hospital, and a native hospital with an outpatients clinic. Whether a private doctor set up practice cannot be established with any certainty.[103]

Disputes between Doctors and the Administration

The position of doctors within the colonial hierarchy and the relationship with its other members was not unambiguous. On the one hand doctors

---

98 In the colonial salary scales doctors ranked as 4b; governors were in the first category, judges of the high court in the second, 'Referenten' in the third, district officers and judges in category 4a; category 4b included doctors and senior civil and construction engineers. *Deutsches Kolonial-Lexikon* I: 85; 459. *Amtsblatt* 1911: 183-4

99 Hahl to RKA 15.4.1909, RKA 5731: 75 ff; 98 ff

100 RKA 5731: 240-44

101 *DKZ* 29 (1912): 251

102 RKA to Hahl 17.12.1912, RKA 5731: 124-5

103 Dr Wendland left the government medical service, but there is some circumstantial evidence suggesting that he opened the first private practice in Rabaul in 1914. See biographical notes in Appendix II.

claimed highest authority in all medical matters and full freedom of action; on the other they were employees of the New Guinea Company and as such under the authority of the administrator, and their first duty was to the interests of the company. Clashes of interest and friction between the local company administrators and doctors were unavoidable. The conflict that arose in Friedrich-Wilhelmshafen between Dr Diesing and the acting administrator, Skopnik, and the station manager, Wandres, in 1897/98 serves to illustrate the type of dispute that could arise which led to the resignation of Diesing after less than one year's service.

Diesing reported Wandres repeatedly to the administrator because of ill-treatment of labourers, but no action was taken. Complaints by Diesing about this state of affairs were apparently considered inappropriate, and insults were traded, leading to a court case in which Diesing was fined. In this strained atmosphere Diesing ordered some Javanese to bring water to the hospital; they refused to do so, knowing exactly who had authority on the station and who had not. Diesing's complaint to the administrator met with the reprimand that it was in any case not Diesing's, but the station manager's job to ensure water at the hospital. The situation became farcical when the administrator insisted on written orders between the three parties. Legitimate demands by the doctor, such as clearing the land around the hospital of long grass, were ignored and led to a further complaint by the doctor. Petty squabbles came to a head when the administrator directly infringed on the doctor's authority and insisted that it was neither at the doctor's nor the station manager's bidding that medical examinations of female labourers were to be carried out; it was a matter of public health and as such to be carried out at the orders of the administrator. At this point Diesing resigned and returned home.[104]

Absurd as the behaviour of all concerned was, it did show up the weaknesses of the system. Principles of authority were involved; the interests of company management and doctors were not identical. A doctor's authority was limited to examining recruits; the decision on a recruit's fitness rested with company management in the person of the station manager. He was, of course, reluctant to hospitalise or repatriate people brought to Kaiser-Wilhelmsland at great expense.[105]

Apart from tensions that arose out of structural problems, newcomers were

104 RKA 2414: 38-39; 47-62
105 Paragraph 4 in 'Verordnung, betreffend die gesundheitliche Kontrolle der als Arbeiter angeworbenen Eingeborenen', dated 19 November 1891, *DKG* 553-5; also New Guinea Company (afterwards NGC) to Auswärtiges Amt [Foreign Office] (afterwards AA) 2.2.1891, RKA 2301: 102

under great psychological and physiological stresses. Their general state of health was weakened by malaria; many may have been adversely affected by quinine; although food supply was adequate, it was a monotonous, nutritionally poor diet, lacking in fresh fruit and vegetables; the number of expatriates was small and social intercourse for weeks at a time was restricted to the few people on the station; alcohol consumption was high if customs returns are any indication: altogether not an environment in which people of disparate backgrounds and with different interests, haphazardly thrown together, could necessarily work together.

With the hand-over of administrative authority to the Reich, doctors were employed by the government and responsible to the governor. Within the structure for government employees there was still room for disagreements, but there seems to have been only one case in which open warfare broke out. As this case highlights a number of aspects, such as the suitability of a particular type of doctor for colonial service, the relations between government employees, and the administrative decision making process, it is worth looking at in some detail.

When Dr Seibert arrived at the beginning of 1905, he considered himself to be well qualified for the work. He had attended a six-week training course at the Institute of Tropical Medicine in Hamburg before he applied for a medical appointment in a colony. He was given to understand that he would be posted to Simpsonhafen (Rabaul), where it was planned to move the central government administration. There he would be responsible for creating an environment fit for human habitation, corresponding to the latest standards set for public health. In order to increase his knowledge of tropical medicine, he worked for about three months at the Institute for Infectious Diseases in Berlin at his own expense. Thus equipped, conscious of his professional status, he was well prepared to meet the challenges. His first job was to replace Dr Wendland in Herbertshöhe during the latter's leave for twelve months, and following that, he was sent to replace Dr Hoffmann in Friedrich-Wilhelmshafen during his home leave. Seibert finally started work in Simpsonhafen in July 1906. For nearly eighteen months he had confronted routine cases of malaria, dysentery, beriberi and tropical ulcers and minor injuries—not quite the type of work for a doctor of his training and leanings.

While at Herbertshöhe he was asked to make a professional assessment of measures needed to make Simpsonhafen a healthy place, at long last an assignment for which his course at the Hamburg institute had prepared him. His long list of recommendations included systematic and continuous quinine prophylaxis and therapy; further clearing and burning off of bush and planting of grass; filling in of water holes along the beach; fitting of all rain water tanks and future wells with tight-fitting lids; setting of roof guttering at much steeper angles so water could run off completely; no planting of coconut palms within designated building areas as they provided breeding ground and shelter for mosquitoes; greatest attention to be paid to water supply; all water to be filtered; all waste products to be removed in closed buckets; all houses built by the government to be constructed to meet the standards set in relation to tropical hygiene and no house to be occupied without certification by the doctor responsible for public health; the construction of a native hospital, a quarantine station, a house for medical orderlies, a house for the doctor, a pharmacy, a hospital for Europeans, a house for nursing sisters (plans and sites for all buildings had already been approved). The recommendations were accepted by the governor, and some minor works were carried out.

A few days after taking up his appointment in Simpsonhafen Seibert wrote another report about the local health conditions and, as nothing happened, followed it up with another missive three weeks later. He pointed out that the slashing and burning of bush had been helpful in temporarily reducing the mosquito plague, but that in general health conditions were appalling because of the large number of people working in Simpsonhafen. However, prospects for creating a healthy environment in Simpsonhafen were good provided his recommendations were all carried out.[106] From what followed it is clear that Seibert expected that immediate steps would be taken on his recommendations. When nothing of the sort happened—and all he was doing was looking after six hundred labourers and twenty Europeans with the well known problems of malaria, dysentery and ulcers—he renewed his campaign early in September 1906. His reports became abusive, laced with accusations of inefficiency and incompetence and wild exaggerations, not endearing him to the administration. In his single-minded fight for the improvement of sanitary conditions, he objected to any other priorities of the administration, such as the building of a school for native children. He lost sight of finances and the lengthy process involved in getting approval for any funding. He seemed to have little understanding of how the government operated, and the strict budget which, in the last instance, was determined by the Reichstag.

There were certainly grounds for Seibert's complaints and they were considered fully justified by the government medical officer in Herbertshöhe, Dr Wendland. There was an urgent need to construct a quarantine station and

106 RKA 5729: 23, 109-110; RKA 5769: 21-26

there were problems with the water supply and sanitation. The lack of sanitary facilities meant that over six hundred people used the surrounding bush for defecation, with the result that food and water were contaminated, and a high incidence of dysentery followed. Krauss, the acting governor, pointed out that even if there were enough latrines, "it would be impossible to make people use them." Therefore, sanitary facilities were built where their use could be somewhat controlled, namely in the hospital. Without consulting Seibert, the administration rented sheds and two small houses from Hernsheim & Co. to be used as a temporary native hospital and accommodation for the doctor and the medical orderly. By spending just over 1000 Mark for cement floors in the two buildings to be used as hospitals, installation of three closets and water tanks, repairs to the water pump, and fencing around the grounds, the government did "all that could be done with the modest means available".[107]

It was a useful excuse for the government to argue that labourers were not using any sanitary facilities; it was a way of avoiding an intractable problem. While traditional sanitary habits of the widely dispersed indigenous population were reasonably safe as long as people were living in their hamlets and villages, they ceased to be so the moment labourers were thrown together into large, close-living groups. The provision of adequate sanitary facilities was therefore a government responsibility, and so was the training of labourers to use these facilities.

It appears that Seibert was never told the real reason why neither the native hospital nor the quarantine station were being built. When he arrived there, a final decision had not been made in Berlin for transferring the administration to Simpsonhafen and until such time as that decision was made, no money would be forthcoming for infrastructures. His very campaign delayed such a decision, for in his zeal to get things done, he approached the Colonial Office directly, and suggested that Simpsonhafen was not a suitable location for a capital after all as, quite apart from serious reservations he now had about it from a public health point of view, there was not enough land available to house Europeans well away from Chinese and native quarters. At a time when the Colonial Office was about to agree to Hahl's proposal for the siting of the administrative centre at the deep harbour in Blanche Bay, a plan he had been nursing along since 1899, Seibert's doubts about the place caused alarm and the Colonial Office called for further reports and expert opinions, not only from Hahl, but also from a naval surveyor and a naval surgeon, and a civil engineer, who was sent from Germany to examine the proposal. All experts agreed that the best

107 RKA 5730: 132-143

harbour in the Bismarck Archipelago was Simpsonhafen, and that the administrative centre of the colony should be located in the shipping and commercial
centre, and that all problems in relation to public health could be solved by
technical means and by the segregation of the races in the new town.[108]

In this last respect Seibert had been successful. In a report submitted shortly before his departure, he reiterated recommendations made over the years
by other doctors in regard to malaria treatment and eradication by saying that
"a fundamental condition is that housing for natives and Chinese is built at
least one kilometre away from European housing."[109] The medical *Referent* in
the Colonial Office, Dr Steudel, fully supported him and ordered that "segregation of European housing from dwellings of natives is to be carried out
strictly. A native hospital, a native prison and barracks for labourers and soldiers in or near a European quarter are a dangerous threat to the health of
Europeans."[110] Quinine prophylaxis as a public health measure, quietly
dropped some years earlier, was now officially abandoned and racial segregation adopted. It was far less demanding of medical services and therefore
cheaper, and easier to apply as a general principle.

Seibert's high expectations of important scientific research were dashed; his
specialised skills were rarely used. Apart from analysing drinking water, he was
fully occupied with the daily routine of a medical practitioner. He was quite
the wrong person for personal contact with patients as he felt only revulsion
at the "hideous fetid ulcers" and the "disgusting skin diseases". In his eager-
ness to solve all problems, he made enemies among administrators. He was much
happier working in a laboratory. As it was, his high-strung nature, his fastidious-
ness, his high sense of duty and consciousness of his status all combined to make
his life very difficult. He suffered considerable ill-health because of dysentery
while he was in New Guinea, and the mental stress caused by his quarrels with
authorities also affected his health. When he left New Guinea his health was
ruined, "a victim of his profession and of science".[111] His experience showed that
there was a wide gap between research and its practical application. He arrived
in the belief that a quinine program and ecological measures would eradicate
malaria; he left convinced that racial segregation was the answer to the malaria
problem for the colonists. He returned to laboratory work in Hamburg.

---

108 RKA 5774: 3-7. There is an interesting parallel here with the choice of Friedrich-
  Wilhelmshafen (Madang) in Kaiser-Wilhelmsland; it was also chosen because of its deep
  water harbour; reservations about health hazards were overruled. See *NKWL* 1897: 16
109 RKA 5770: 131
110 RKA 5774: 24
111 RKA 5730: 134; RKA 5769: 129

The episode also says something about the administration. Obviously there was petty-mindedness, for it appears that Seibert was not told that the construction of Rabaul had not yet been approved by Berlin. He endeared himself to nobody when he could show up incompetence and negligence.[112] Yet the administration could not be blamed entirely if Seibert's research skills could not be properly used in New Guinea. While funds were restricted, the administration saw its first responsibility as providing basic medical services; research work had to be postponed until more staff and funds for better facilities were available. Seibert was an extreme example of the wrong person to be sent to the colonies. Other doctors, with similar qualifications but fewer illusions, coped with similar frustrations. Nevertheless, it raises also the question whether a doctor was necessarily the best person to undertake the work that had to be done in New Guinea at that time. Limited resources might have been more usefully invested in medical orderlies and nursing sisters who could cope with the routine nature of most of the work in hospitals or outstations without a doctor.

Doctors' Employment Record

The employment record of doctors over the 30-year period shows clearly that an improvement of general conditions (which included the transfer of the colony's centre from mainland New Guinea to the Bismarck Archipelago) together with regular quinine prophylaxis and a build-up of immunity against malaria began to make German New Guinea a viable place of residence not only for doctors but also other colonists.

For the period 1885 to 1901 the record of employing doctors for Kaiser-Wilhelmsland was disastrous. In sixteen years the New Guinea Company had contracts for two or three year periods with fifteen doctors, and employed another three on a temporary basis to fill in while awaiting the new appointee. Of the fifteen doctors, only three—Schellong, Wendland and Dempwolff—remained for the full period of their contract. Two died while working in Kaiser-Wilhelmsland, Weinland in 1891, and Emmerling in 1893. At least three left because of ill health (Hagen, Hintze and Schlafke), and one was dismissed (Herrmann). The reasons for the other five early departures cannot be established for certain; some may have left for health reasons, others because of disagreements with company management, and perhaps most of them because of a combination of both.

---

112 He cited as an example that, despite his repeated remonstrations, a badly needed new autoclave was left sitting in Herbertshöhe for nine months after arrival from Germany before it was transported to Simpsonhafen, only to be damaged during the short trip. RKA 5769: 125

The first government medical officer in Kaiser-Wilhelmsland was Dr Hoffmann who worked in Friedrich-Wilhelmshafen from August 1902 to mid-1910 (from where he transferred to Kaewieng). His successor, Dr Liesegang, was there from mid-1910 until his repatriation by the Australian authorities.

In the Bismarck Archipelago a government medical officer for Herberts-höhe was approved in the 1901 budget. However, budget requests for the construction of a government native hospital in Herbertshöhe were not approved. This lack led directly to delay and eventual abandonment of work on malaria research. The contract of the New Guinea Company doctor in Herbertshöhe, Dr Fuhrmann, expired on 7 February 1902,[113] two months after Wendland, the new government appointee, was to take up his job in Herbertshöhe. The government needed accommodation in a native hospital for its labour force; as it had no hospital of its own, it was forced to use the facilities of the company hospital. The company in turn was no longer keen on appointing its own doctor for Herbertshöhe, arguing that the government medical officer should take over the care of all labourers as part of his duties in Herbertshöhe. With the imminent departure of Fuhrmann, the company's labourers could not be left without medical services. The New Guinea Company was quick to take advantage of the appointment of a government medical officer and submitted a proposal to the Colonial Department whereby the company would pay an agreed fee to the government for Wendland's services. The administration could only accept this proposal; funds for its own native hospital would be available in the next budget at the earliest, and it could not risk having no accommodation for sick recruits and labourers.[114] This meant that Wendland was involved in the malaria testing program for only about two months; after that, for all practical purposes, the situation remained as it had been—there was just one doctor in Herbertshöhe and he was busy with the routine day-to-day practice.

Plans for a government medical service had been different. Apart from the care of people in government employ it was intended that, the service carry out malaria research. Professor Koch, who undertook such research in Kaiser-Wilhelmsland, the Bismarck Archipelago, and parts of the Island Territory from late 1899 to mid-1900, had recommended that his malaria eradication program be continued. To this end, as a special project, Dr Dempwolff was sent to the colony and he spent nearly two years in Kaiser-Wilhelmsland and the Bismarck Archipelago.[115] In addition, the government medical officer for

113 RKA 5729: 72
114 Hahl to RKA 10.5.1902, RKA 5729: 90-2
115 O. Dempwolff, 'Bericht über eine Malaria-Expedition nach Deutsch-Neu-Guinea', *Zeitschrift für Hygiene und Infektionskrankheiten* 47 (1904): 81-132

Herbertshöhe was to be trained in bacteriology so that he could also work on malaria programs. When this plan faltered because of the practical demands in the colony, Governor Hahl was philosophical about the situation—while there was only one hospital in Herbertshöhe there was no point in having two doctors in the cramped and badly equipped New Guinea Company hospital. Any scientific work a doctor might be able to do would have to be restricted to the immediate surroundings of Herbertshöhe, and postponed in other areas. There was in any case the problem that while there was no motor vessel, trips to the more distant areas of New Britain and the islands would mean a doctor's lengthy absence, which was undesirable, considering the number of Europeans residing in Herbertshöhe.[116]

The employment of government medical officers roughly coincided with new knowledge about a proper dosage of quinine for malaria prophylaxis and doctors stayed on longer after the turn of the century if they were able to take quinine regularly without suffering side effects, and to build up malaria immunity. It is notable though that, during his first tour in Kaiser-Wilhelmsland from 1894 to 1897, Wendland experimented on himself by taking one gram of quinine weekly. This did not fully protect him from malaria, but he had far fewer attacks than other Europeans who took quinine only therapeutically. On his return from home leave he worked at Herbertshöhe for nineteen months without taking any quinine before he had the first malaria attack, and after quinine therapy, he remained again malaria-free.[117] Doctors set an example for quinine prophylaxis. When he first arrived in Friedrich-Wilhelmshafen, Hoffmann took 1 gram of quinine every fifth day. While this did not entirely prevent light malaria attacks in the first three months, after that time he had attacks only if he did not take quinine regularly, and after about a year in the colony he found that a weekly intake of this dosage was sufficient.[118] His successor, Liesegang, avoided malaria by taking quinine according to Nocht's method: every fourth day he took one gram of quinine hydrochloride in five doses of 0.2 gram each, the first dose before dinner in the evening, the second that same night before going to bed, the third the next morning on an empty stomach, the fourth and fifth doses the same as the night before.[119] Wick, who began his malaria prophylaxis the day he arrived in Herbertshöhe, also remained malaria-free.[120]

116 RKA 5729: 142-43

117 W. Wendland, 'Ueber Chininprophylaxe in Neuguinea', *ASTH* 10 (1904): 431-54

118 MB 1903/4: 211-12

119 MB 1910/11: 633-34

120 W. Wick, 'Physiologische Studien zur Akklimatisation an die Tropen', *ASTH* 14 (1910): 650-16

It is therefore not surprising that the employment record of all doctors was very good and most government medical officers stayed in the colony for a number of years. Wendland could look back on sixteen years in German New Guinea (nearly four with the company in Kaiser-Wilhelmsland, and over twelve years as government medical officer in Herbertshöhe/Rabaul). Hoffmann had had nearly twelve years of practice in German New Guinea when he returned permanently to Germany early in 1914; Runge had worked there for eight years when war broke out, and Wick six years.

There were other reasons why doctors began to make work in German New Guinea a career. Friction with company management was no longer a constant feature of life. If problems arose, the doctor was responsible to the governor, not to company management. Doctors were no longer isolated professionally and socially. Professionally they were part of a developing medical speciality, tropical medicine, which was gaining increasing importance and recognition in medical circles; they were members of a professional association, the German Society of Tropical Medicine; working conditions were generally improving as facilities such as well equipped hospitals were built. As the European population increased, so did the social circle; housing improved and they were able to bring families with them to German New Guinea; together with their wives, doctors were leading members of the colonial society; in the Rabaul Club they were playing their part;[121] in brief, they were involved in the creation of a microcosm of German middle-class life and in building a colony. As government employees they had employment and retirement security. Paid home leave after three years in the colony and further professional training while in Germany were other attractive features of government employment. Altogether, some ten years after the Reich took over the administration of German New Guinea, life there started to look good for a doctor.

The gradual changes in the situation of doctors, characterised by improved health and general living conditions, were paralleled by the experiences of all Europeans who ventured to the colony. Their health and ill health is the topic of the next chapter.

---

121 Dr Wick and his wife gave well attended piano and violin recitals at the Rabaul Club. The concert program for the opening concert of the Rabaul Club in March 1910 included an amateur quartet playing Schubert, Handel and Beethoven. *Amtsblatt* 1910: 51 and 63. Mrs

2

THE EUROPEANS

When it comes to Europeans, the best is barely good enough.[1]

In this chapter I discuss the medical problems encountered by Europeans in German New Guinea and the measures taken to protect their health. The newcomers were all affected by diseases endemic in the colony; in turn they brought in new diseases which had a serious impact on the native population. These are discussed in the first part of this chapter; the second part deals with infrastructure necessary to maintain the health of Europeans—medical services, hospitals, nurses, housing and public works.

The effect of the climate in New Guinea was vastly underestimated, and warnings were ignored by enthusiastic entrepreneurs who founded the New Guinea Company. When evidence of this danger mounted, it was played down, much to the later chagrin of many an enterprising but ignorant company employee. Yet the poor state of health meant not only individual suffering and premature deaths, but also considerable cost to the company and to the economic development of the colony.

Although medical records for Kaiser-Wilhelmsland during the company period are incomplete and inconsistent, it is clear that malaria was the overwhelming health problem until the turn of the century, and it remained ever-present in the life of all settlers afterwards. Analyses of malaria from the early

Wick played an active part in the Women's League and became its president following the departure of Mrs. Hahl.

days to the turn of the century have been made by Ewers and by Jackman[2] and need not be repeated here. I shall look briefly at malaria in the period after 1900 and at some other health problems experienced by the colonists, and then consider the attempts of administrations and doctors to combat disease and maintain or improve the health of newcomers.

The basis of the health care system in Germany were hospitals and sanatoria and they proliferated there in the 1880s and '90s.[3] The metropolitan system served as the model for the colonies, which is to say that in New Guinea hospitals were seen as an essential part of the infrastructure of the colony, both as the base for a doctor, and a place for nursing the sick. As the number of Europeans grew, so did the need for hospitals. While their establishment became the focus for political pressure, hospitals also became a centre for social interaction. The cost of hospitals—construction and running costs—was out of proportion to the small number of patients, or the limited number of people entitled to use them. Because of the size of the colony and its widely dispersed European centres, there were strong pressures to build a hospital in each centre. Closely connected to good overall conditions for settlers were housing and sanitation, and I touch on these briefly.

The need to ensure and promote the health and well being of settlers guided decisions on providing medical services and infrastructures but, as time went by, the need to maintain the integrity of the European race, based on notions of racial hygiene, also began to influence decision-making.

HEALTH AND ILL HEALTH

Kaiser-Wilhelmsland: Morbidity and Mortality

The year 1891 was undoubtedly the nadir of German colonisation in New Guinea; the disastrous health situation in Finschhafen early in 1891, when many died, and which led to the evacuation of the settlement, has been taken up by

1 Hahl to Dr Danneil on selecting sites for housing and hospitals for Europeans. PNG Archives G255/892: 12

2 W.H. Ewers, 'Malaria in the early years of German New Guinea', *Journal of the Papua and New Guinea Society* 6.1 (1972): 3-30. H.J. Jackman, '*Nunquam otiosus* and the two Ottos: Malaria in German New Guinea', in B.G. Burton-Bradley ed., A *History of Medicine in Papua New Guinea*, (Kingsgrove, NSW: Australasian Medical Publishing Co. Ltd., 1990) 119-149

other writers, and there is no need for reiteration.[4] However, the move to Stephansort, a company plantation settlement fifteen kilometres south of the Gogol River, and then to Friedrich-Wilhelmshafen, did not bring much respite, for influenza had also reached New Guinea "on its trip around the world" in the early 1890s[5] and affected Europeans, the labour force and the local population alike.[6] It is possible that some of the fifteen or more people who died in Finschhafen at the beginning of 1891 of a particularly virulent malaria had been weakened by influenza. Influenza certainly affected many towards the end of 1891, and the situation was precarious as Imperial Commissioner Rose's report to Chancellor Caprivi showed. Table 1 (below) depicts the situation on 17 December 1891 in the Friedrich-Wilhelmshafen area[7].

Of the thirty-two sick, two died within days, and two others returned to Germany. Despite the presence of two nursing sisters in Friedrich-Wilhelmshafen from June 1891 on, the high death rate early in the year had brought about a change in policy. Rather than wait for an improvement in their condition, patients were sent to the Bismarck Archipelago or to Singapore to recuperate, or, if unlikely to recover under the given conditions, repatriated. These figures relate only to men in the employ of the company. Of the thirty-two patients listed, twenty were sent aboard the *Ysabel* to the Bismarck

Table 1
Morbidity in Friedrich-Wilhelmshafen on 17 December 1891

Station	Total healthy	Total	Malaria	Influenza	Total sick
Stephansort	16	7	4	5	9
Friedrich-Wilhelmshafen	16	8	2	6	8
Jomba	5	3	2	0	2
Gorima	7	3	2	2	4
Erima	4	1	2	1	3
Constantinhafen	2	1	1	0	1
S.S. *Ysabel*	6	1	2	3	5
Total	**56**	**24**	**15**	**17**	**32**

3   From around 141,000 hospital beds in 1876, the numbers grew to 370,000 by 1900. Weindling 19

4   The evacuation of Finschhafen features in Ewers, 'Malaria in the early years'; Jackmann, 'Malaria in German New Guinea'; also Stewart Firth, *New Guinea under the Germans* (Melbourne: Melbourne UP 1982) 31

5   *NKWL* 1890: 86-7; also Rose RKA 6512: 76

6   This outbreak was possibly part of the 1889-93 pandemic which spread across Europe from Russia and reached England in early 1890, with 'peak waves' in January 1890, May 1891,

Archipelago:[8] the ship was so overloaded that it could hardly leave port.[9] Those left in Friedrich-Wilhelmshafen were despondent; Sister Hertzer was very weak, hardly able to look after the remaining patients.[10]

There was no repetition of the 1891 crisis but health conditions remained precarious because of the prevailing malaria. Doctors calculated that on average each European came down with malaria every tenth day in Stephansort and every eighth day in Friedrich-Wilhelmshafen.[11] It is no wonder that malaria research carried out by Professor Koch in Stephansort raised high hopes that at long last a method was in the offing to combat this ubiquitous ailment. While it had been known for a long time that quinine was helpful against malaria, dosage and frequency of intake were haphazard with the result that doses insufficient to have much effect were taken, or too large a dosage which could lead to blackwater fever, a type of often fatal quinine poisoning. Koch's studies in Stephansort led him to establishing an effective dosage schedule to prevent a malaria relapse, and during his stay there was a remarkable reduction in the incidence of malaria. Perhaps of greater importance was his finding that young children suffer most from malaria and that over time a person develops immunity to malaria through regular exposure to infection.

But, despite Koch's success in establishing a quinine schedule, malaria continued to dominate. In 1903/04, when sixteen to twenty Europeans were based in Friedrich-Wilhelmshafen, Dr Hoffmann treated forty-seven malaria cases: on average a person in Friedrich-Wilhelmshafen had at least two attacks during the year severe enough to warrant medical attention. Moreover, as Hoffmann pointed out, the situation was similar in the rest of Kaiser-Wilhelmsland[12], except that no doctor was readily available. However, by 1910, when 234 Europeans lived in the Friedrich-Wilhelmshafen region, there were only fourteen cases of malaria and one of blackwater fever, and malaria had "lost some of its terror".[13] The swamps on which Friedrich-Wilhelmshafen was built had been filled in over a number of years, with very beneficial results.[14]

If regular quinine intake was not adopted by all, neither were other recognised measures for combating malaria. In Hoffmann's view Koch's method of

January 1892 and December 1893. Macfarlane Burnett, *Natural History of Infectious Diseases* (Cambridge: CUP 1953, 2nd ed.) 279

7   Rose to Chancellor von Caprivi 24.12.1891, RKA 2980
8   Diary of Auguste Hertzer, 17 December 1891 (excerpts). Archives Robert-Koch-Institut
9   Rose to Chancellor von Caprivi 24.12.1891, RKA 2980: 200-1
10   Hertzer diary, 17 December 1891
11   Wendland and Dempwolff reports for April to October 1896. *NKWL* 1896

screening the whole population and identifying all parasite carriers and then treating them with quinine for a considerable length of time was simply not practicable in Kaiser-Wilhelmsland. Given the large number of personnel needed to carry out blood tests and supervise the proper ingestion of quinine in the dispersed population—native and colonists—the cost was prohibitive. Avoiding contact with mosquitoes through complete screening of all houses was also expensive and in practice an unrealistic approach, bound to fail because of shortcomings on the part of settlers. They rarely bothered to ensure that mosquito nets were in good order and it was therefore unlikely that they would maintain screens properly. Furthermore, screening of doors and windows was unacceptable to most people as this inhibited the free flow of air. The destruction of breeding places, the so-called "English method"[15], could not be implemented as it was unsuitable for local conditions, and was really useful only in an urban setting. The only way to reducing the number and intensity of malaria relapses that Hoffmann could see was consistent and regular individual quinine prophylaxis. He regretted this method was not compulsory but depended on "discernment and good will".[16] These two qualities were apparently scarce, both in New Guinea and in other German colonies, among settlers, and among government employees. The question of compulsory quinine prophylaxis for all Government employees in the colonies was discussed in Berlin at a meeting of colonial doctors and officials from the Colonial Department. It was decided that, although very desirable, it was not possible to implement and in place of compulsion there should be instruction and exhortation.[17] It is notable that so soon after malaria eradication seemed promised, a compulsory quininisation program was seen as unenforceable and unrealistic; instead, malaria had become accepted as part of the way of German colonial life. For New Guinea it meant the constant loss of staff and their replacement by inexperienced personnel. Rose despaired of any progress in the colony in 1891[18]; fifteen years later Governor Hahl was more optimistic, but conceded that malaria imposed a "severe handicap to development".[19]

Table 2 (page 54) analyses company personnel movements from 1885-1898. The figures are only approximate, but give a picture of the high staff turnover and the length of time New Guinea Company employees stayed

12   MB 1903/04: 206
13   MB 1910/11: 633
14   MB 1911/12: 491
15   So called because it was recommended by Ronald Ross, the first to demonstrate that the mosquito is responsible for the transmission of malaria.
16   MB 1903/04: 208-10

in the colony.[20] For this analysis, a three-year contract is assumed.[21]

With one in five Europeans dying up to 1898, death rates were high indeed, particularly as most people were aged between twenty and thirty-five.[22] The 1890 arrivals were by far the least fortunate—they were the group most affected by the virulent malaria outbreak early in 1891 and influenza. The figure of seventeen deaths does not include children, of whom at least two died.[23]

One way of dealing with malaria and its effects was to leave the country. Many did so in the early days, and it remained a last resort throughout the German period. The table indicates that more than one third left the colony before completing their contract. The 1892 cohort had a particularly high rate of early departures with nine leaving within one year and two within two years. The years 1891 to 1893 have a high number of 'unknown'; it is probably safe to assume that many of these took fright and left Kaiser-

Table 2
Personnel movements 1885–1898

Year arrived	Total arrivals	Deaths	Left w/in 1 year	Left w/in 1–2 yrs	Completed contract	Renewed contract	Unknown
1885	4	0	0	0	3	0	1
1886	27	6	6	6	5	1	3
1887	27	7	3	1	4	4	8
1888	28	7	8	3	2	3	5
1889	6	2	1	0	2	1	0
1890	33	17	6	0	1	3	6
1891	31	1	4	7	1	5	13
1892	22	1	9	2	4	0	6
1893	22	1	6	2	0	3	10
1894	13	3	0	5	1	2	2
1895	12	2	4	4	0	0	2
1896	6	1	1	1	2	0	1
1897	12	1	8	2	n/a	n/a	1
1898	17	3	1	n/a	n/a	n/a	13
Total	260	52	57	33	25	22	71

17   *DKB* 14 (1903): 260

18   Rose to Chancellor von Caprivi 24.12.1891, RKA 2980: 195 ff

19   AR 1907/08: 280

20   Because personnel files of the NGC no longer exist, it is not possible fully to reconstruct personnel statistics. Not all staff movements were reported, nor are there clear indications whether an employee was accompanied by his family, except in the case of Administrator von Schleinitz. The figures have been calculated from reports in *NKWL*, Annual Reports, and Colonial Office files. Shipping crews are not included in these calculations.

21   "Left before completion of contract" does not tell us anything about the length of contract. Indications are that not all employees were engaged for the same length of time; that there were some 2-year contracts (such as Schellong), but also 3-year contracts.

Wilhelmsland in a hurry. Of the 1898 arrivals many may have stayed on, but they cannot be identified.

The New Guinea Company was very careful in reporting the situation in Kaiser-Wilhelmsland. The emphasis was on achievements, exploration, and description of the country. Any small success or apparent success was reported in full, but set-backs were played down. By not reporting all staff movements it was not obvious just how many people returned early. The low morale of the staff and the hopelessness of the situation as described in Hertzer's diary were, naturally, not published in company's organ, the *Nachrichten von Kaiser-Wilhelmsland*; nor was the fact that most people—black and white—suffered from fever daily, as she did.[24] However, the company had to admit that in just over four years, some thirteen Europeans (19% of employees) based in Friedrich-Wilhelmshafen had left the company before completing their contract.[25] Expectations that people who had been working in a tropical country would be inured to the rigours of New Guinea proved utterly false also. Tobacco planters recruited in the Dutch East Indies succumbed to malaria as readily as all others.

Repatriation on health grounds still occurred after 1900 but nowhere to the same extent as before. "Chronic malaria" or "malaria with complications" more often than not were the grounds on which a person was sent back to Germany. For example, in 1905 three New Guinea Company employees were sent back to Germany: one was a case of malaria with complications, the second neurasthenia complicated by malaria, the third because of general physical disposition which made him unsuitable to live in a tropical climate; in 1908 one recent arrival was repatriated because of blackwater fever and another because of chronic malaria and chronic morphinism.[26]

There were one hundred and thirty known deaths of Europeans in Kaiser-Wilhelmsland during the German period.[27] Before looking at the table a few words of caution, the first being that there is no claim to completeness and accuracy. Early records in particular are incomplete, diagnosis was not always made by a doctor and, what is more important, usually a single or the primary cause of death was recorded. (If multiple causes were listed, only the first cause was counted in order to simplify the table.) Nevertheless, Table 3 gives an indication of general trends. The breakdown is as follows (rounded percentage figures):

22 Dempwolff, for instance, makes the point that Europeans under his care were mostly in their twenties. Dempwolff, 'Aerztliche Erfahrungen' 136

23 For example, one of General Manager Wissmann's children died.

24 Hertzer diary, 11 December 1891

Table 3
Cause of death of Europeans, Kaiser-Wilhelmsland 1886-1914

Cause of death	Number	Per cent
malaria and/or blackwater fever	74	57
accidental deaths	12	9
homicide	11	8
influenza, pneumonia, pleurisy	6	5
tuberculosis	4	3
appendicitis, peritonitis	2	2
dysentery	2	2
heart disease	4	3
maternal death, stillbirth	2	2
miscellaneous	7	5
unknown	6	5

With fifty-seven per cent of deaths due to malaria and/or blackwater fever, these were undoubtedly the main cause of death in Kaiser-Wilhelmsland during the German period.

If the number of total deaths is broken down to the period to the end of 1899, there were seventy-seven deaths for that period of which forty-nine, or sixty-four per cent belong into the malaria/blackwater category. In the period after the introduction of quinine there were fifty-three deaths, of which twenty-four or forty-five per cent were malarial. This suggests a decrease in malarial deaths of nearly twenty per cent after the introduction of quinine. However, the category 'unknown' creates an obstacle in this simple arithmetic. But even if this is taken into account, the figures would be sixty-five percent for the early period and fifty-five per cent for the later period, indicating a reduction in malarial deaths of about ten percent. In view of the foregoing discussion of the difficulties encountered in persuading colonists to follow Koch's quinine schedule, we are left wondering whether the decrease was due to a quinine regimen or whether settlers started to acquire a certain degree of immunity. The extent to which many of the other listed causes, such as heart disease, delirium, and mental disturbance, were connected with malaria remains another open question. Furthermore, we do not know whether deaths attributable to malaria occurred following repatriation.

Bismarck Archipelago: Morbidity and Mortality

From 1887 to 1914, around two hundred and twelve Europeans[28] died in the Bismarck Archipelago administrative district. Causes of death are set out

25   NKWL 1896: 22

Table 4
Cause of death of Europeans, Bismarck Archipelago 1886-1914

Cause of death	Number	Per cent
malaria and blackwater fever	44	21
homicide	48	23
tuberculosis	14	7
accidental deaths	16	8
heart failure/disease	9	4
dysentery	9	4
pneumonia	7	3
suicide	9	4
alcoholism and liver cirrhosis	8	4
maternal deaths, stillbirth	7	3
meningitis, encephalitis	2	1
typhus	4	2
appendicitis, peritonitis	3	1
miscellaneous	8	4
unknown	24	11

in Table 4 (percentage figures rounded).

About one in five deaths were due to malaria and blackwater fever, a rate considerably lower than in Kaiser-Wilhelmsland, where they accounted for nearly three out of five deaths. However, the figures have to be approached with caution, as the diagnoses are mostly single-cause, and malaria should not be underestimated as a contributing factor. With about 8 per cent of deaths due to tuberculosis, there was concern from a public health point of view. Around one in six deaths was due to fatal encounters with natives. Nine people died of dysentery, a figure which suggests that water supply and sanitation were not adequate even for newcomers.[29]

Unlike in Kaiser-Wilhelmsland, where medical services were established first and foremost for the colonists, in the Bismarck Archipelago the New Guinea Company brought in the first medical orderly in 1890 to take care of labour recruits in the newly established labour depot in Herbertshöhe.[30] A medical orderly, but no doctor, was stationed at Herbertshöhe for the next five years until Dr Danneil was appointed as company medical officer, taking up work there in January 1896. At this stage the company was expanding its cotton plantations, which required a much larger labour force. Together with labourers from other plantations a large enough population pool was created

26   MB 1905/06: 278; MB 1908/09: 386-9
27   See list of deaths of Europeans in Appendix V. List compiled from medical reports, annual reports, *NKWL*, RKA files and other literature.

to warrant the presence of a doctor. Danneil took up his appointment with the understanding that all other firms on the Gazelle Peninsula and the Catholic and Methodist Missions would also contract his services, ensuring an adequate income. However, the firms of Forsayth & Company and Hernsheim & Company refused to subscribe. They may well have decided that they had managed without a resident doctor for many years and would continue to do so, and ask for his services only if needed. For the doctor it meant an income of some 3800 Mark lower than expected.[31]

During Dr Danneil's term at Herbertshöhe (January 1896 to January 1899) he had few European patients. There were reports of cases of malaria and some of dysentery. As officer in charge of public health (*Sanitätspolizei*), one of his early jobs was a check on the three water supply sources: rain water in tanks, wells not far from the beach, and two springs. Although quantity was sufficient, Danneil was not so sure about the quality, as he lacked the technical means to examine water properly. He was confident though that bacterial pollution was unlikely as the wells were deep and the springs were fed through thick layers of soil masses which in both cases should filter out all micro-organisms.[32] However, recurrent outbreaks of dysentery forced him to revise his judgement within a year.[33]

In cases of malaria, people sought Danneil's help only if the attack was severe.[34] This pattern of illness among settlers persisted until early 1900, when an outbreak of influenza seriously affected many, although none fatally.[35] This was followed by an increase in the incidence and severity of malaria on the Gazelle Peninsula. By that time Professor Koch had visited New Guinea and given instructions on the regular use of quinine, instructions which were more or less ignored. In the first medical report following Koch's visit, Dr Fuhrmann lamented that "the incidence of malaria could be reduced considerably if only people could be persuaded to keep up Koch's quinine therapy."[36]

As in Kaiser-Wilhelmsland, the crux of the matter on the Gazelle Peninsula was how to persuade people to take quinine regularly and in sufficient quantity. One doctor after another battled with this problem. There was a long-running debate among doctors and research scientists on the most efficacious and least disagreeable method of intake.[37] The public was not

28 See list of deaths of Europeans in Appendix V.
29 This list does not of course take into account those who died as a consequence of illness after leaving the colony.
30 AR 1889-90: 52
31 RKA 2986: 56-57
32 *NKWL* 1897: 37
33 *NKWL* 1898: 35-6
34 *NKWL* 1897: 37
35 *AR NGC* 1899/1900: 10, RKA 2419

interested in these debates: a certain amount of malaria was preferable to regular doses of quinine with its unpleasant side effects. Dr Dempwolff, sent to
Kaiser-Wilhelmsland to work further on malaria eradication, was ordered to
take up malaria investigations in the Gazelle Peninsula in mid-1902 following serious cases of malaria and blackwater fever in the Herbertshöhe area.[38]
He noted that "the local people [meaning the colonists] are of the opinion
that it is quite healthy enough here." Resident Germans regarded it as an
affront to their local doctor, Wendland, that malaria research was being
undertaken in the area[39]—an indication that they had not quite the same perception as doctors. For them it had become part of the way of life, rather
than a serious medical problem.

A survey among settlers on the Gazelle Peninsula by Wendland[40]
revealed the highly individual approach most took to quinine prophylaxis.
Of the forty-one respondents, only eight took the dose prescribed by
Koch, that is, 1 gram every ninth and tenth day. Of the others, thirty-one
took doses varying from half a gram to one gram, at intervals of one week
to two weeks; two took quinine only during a malaria attack. A small
dosage was perceived by most as sufficient since fever attacks were fewer
and milder than in pre-prophylaxis days. Numerous rather unpleasant side
effects—ringing in the ears, temporary deafness, severe headaches, nausea,
diarrhoea—were no encouragement to carry out the prescribed regimen.
Wendland was not persuaded that side effects were as severe as his patients
reported; he himself had no difficulty in taking quinine regularly. Some
long-term residents, such as Bishop Couppé from the Sacred Heart Mission,
could defy Koch's prescription with impunity—a weekly dose of half a gram
of quinine kept him virtually free of malaria.

As the European population in the Herbertshöhe/Rabaul area grew, so
did the number seeking medical attention: government employees and their
families, members of the Catholic and the Methodist missions, settlers and
planters and their families, employees of the plantation and trading companies, traders, and people in transit, mainly from merchant and naval ships,
and (later) the German postal steamer. Therefore, the number of
Europeans—which included "half-Samoans" and Japanese—consulting a

---

36 Denkschrift, Aktenstück 437, *Stenographische Berichte der Verhandlungen des Reichstags,*
   1900/01 (10. Legislaturperiode, 2. Session) 5. Anlegeband, 3096
37 Nocht's method became accepted by doctors in German New Guinea as the most appropriate one.
38 Denkschrift, Anlage Aktenstück 54, *Stenographische Berichte der Verhandlungen des Reichstags,*
   1903/04 (11. Legislaturperiode, 2. Session) 1. Anlegeband, 394-8. Dr Hahl, the acting gov-

doctor and listed in statistics, did not correspond to census figures.

The morbidity statistics listed all Europeans who received medical treatment either in the hospital, the polyclinic, or at home. On average per year, fourteen patients were from naval ships' crews, and five were visitors or people in transit. Rabaul was an important centre for treating naval crews for whom facilities on board ship were inadequate. In later years, a few patients came from New Ireland. This means that the number of Europeans treated is somewhat inflated by non-residents. However, it is clear from the commentaries to the statistics that cases of typhus were all from ships' crews.[41] Other comments suggest that malaria, venereal disease and severe injuries were the most common grounds for people in transit or members of ships' crews obtaining medical treatment.

Another factor likely to distort morbidity figures was the availability of a doctor. If a doctor was within reasonably easy reach, people would consult him; if not, they managed without. Morbidity statistics have to be read with some care, thus those for the year 1911/12 seem to indicate that Friedrich-Wilhelmshafen was healthier than Rabaul, when in fact the opposite was true. In the Friedrich-Wilhelmshafen district 234 Europeans were registered, of whom sixty-six consulted a doctor, a morbidity rate of 28.5 per cent. In Rabaul, a district with 385 Europeans, 480 cases were listed,[42] a morbidity rate of 12 per cent for the district.[43] (Herbertshöhe/Rabaul district morbidity statistics are in Appendix VI.)

As Table 5 shows malaria remained the dominant cause of illness in the Herbertshöhe/Rabaul district. With around four out of ten people consulting

Table 5
Malaria incidence in the Rabaul district 1903–1911

Year	Total Patients	Malaria Patients	Percentage
1903	370	152	41
1904	259	106	41
1905	263	105	40
1906	305	108	35
1907	275	110	40
1908	359	100	28
1909	406	93	23
1910	478	127	26
1911	515	98	19

ernor, was one of the people suffering a lot from malaria during the early part of the year and he had a near fatal attack of blackwater fever.

39   Dempwolff to Koch, private letter of 23.9.1902. Archives Robert-Koch-Institut
40   Wendland, 'Ueber Chininprophylaxe in Neuguinea', *ASTH* 10 (1904): 431-54

a doctor because of malaria in the years 1903-7, the incidence remained remarkably steady. With a drop to about three out of ten in 1908, and then about two out of ten in 1909, doctors were optimistic that malaria control was becoming effective. In Dr Born's view, malaria in Herbertshöhe was "no more serious than a heavy cold in Germany."[44] However, it needs to be remembered that the statistics show only patients who sought medical treatment; that is, only the more severe attacks are reflected.

In Simpsonhafen (Rabaul) the situation differed greatly; there work began in 1903 on infrastructure for Norddeutscher Lloyd. In many respects the story was similar to that in Kaiser-Wilhelmsland when stations were first set up. Clearing work created new anopheles breeding places; stretches of swampy ground along the harbour's edge were not filled in promptly; large numbers of newly arrived labourers were crammed together in poorly constructed barracks without sanitation; Europeans lived in nearly as much squalor as labourers. It was an ideal situation for malaria and dysentery. Yet, as Sister Hertzer pointed out, despite the high malaria incidence among recent arrivals, there had been not one malaria death in six months among either European or Chinese in Simpsonhafen, a striking contrast to the situation ten to fifteen years earlier in Kaiser-Wilhelmsland.[45] In her experience, there was no comparison between the virulence of malaria in Kaiser-Wilhelmsland and on the Gazelle Peninsula and therefore the malaria danger in the Bismarck Archipelago should not be overemphasised.

Doctors also attempted to bring about a reduction in malaria through public works and education. With a water shortage at Namanula during an exceptionally dry period in 1910, when a reduction in malaria could be expected, it increased. It turned out that householders were neglectful: empty water tanks were not properly sealed and contained enough damp residue to provide mosquito breeding grounds; empty food tins were thrown under bushes close to houses or into ravines and harboured large numbers of larvae.[46] It was a long and hard battle for doctors to educate the population on the importance of simple and sensible hygienic measures by individual households. However, it was equally difficult to persuade the government that swampy grounds and puddles at Simpsonhafen had to be filled in properly before further construction. The meagre means available for public works of that nature meant slow progress in clearing and filling in Rabaul and

41 In 1907 11 typhus cases were hospitalised from the *Planet* (MB 1907/08: 417-8); 5 in 1910 from the *Cormoran* (MB 1910/11: 636)

42 Total cases 515 less non-residents

43 MB 1911/12: 506-7

44 RKA 5771: 146

Namanula. Even when such work had been done, very often within a matter of weeks the area was overgrown again, as not enough labourers were made available to keep these areas clean.[47] Hahl's response to the unsatisfactory situation was that a transfer of government offices and personnel to Rabaul could not depend on completion of public works—until funds were available, existing conditions had to be accepted.[48] Malaria incidence during the wet season therefore continued at about the same level for years. In the first quarter of 1913, for example, of the seventy-five Europeans treated by a doctor, twenty-three (30%) suffered from malaria.[49] This percentage is similar to the one for the same quarter in 1909, when eighteen of the sixty Europeans were treated for malaria.[50] This figure compared with around 7.5 per cent of all patients in the drier second quarter of 1913,[51] or 15 per cent in the second quarter of 1909.[52] By the beginning of 1914 it could be said that Europeans in Rabaul suffered less from malaria during the dry period than in the earlier years, but the incidence remained steady during the wet season, the result, according to Dr Wick, of inadequate public works.[53]

In an attempt to limit the risks of illness in the tropics the Colonial Department tried to weed out people who were likely to suffer health problems, and regulations were issued in 1902 on the required standard of health of candidates for government colonial service. According to these regulations, the best age for acclimatisation was between twenty-three and thirty. Persons with certain health problems such as nervous conditions of all types, sleeplessness, a tendency to get greatly upset about minor matters, stomach problems, deafness and ear diseases, repeated attacks of rheumatism, kidney disease, pulmonary tuberculosis, venereal disease, habitual heavy drinking and/or smoking, and morphine addiction were not suited to service in the tropics. As part of the medical examination a candidate had to take 1 gram of quinine hydrochlorate to test for any reactions. If other than "slight ringing" in the ear occurred, the person was not fit for tropical service. The Colonial Department also issued instructions on clothing, nutrition, general life style to ensure good health, and tropical diseases, with special emphasis on malaria and venereal disease. The crucial importance of good water was highlighted,

45 Hertzer's report to the Governor on her malaria eradication program in Blanche Bay for the period September to December 1903. Archives Robert-Koch-Institut
46 Wick quarterly report 1.4.-30.6.1910, RKA 5772: 10-2
47 Wick quarterly report 1.10.-31.12.1910, RKA 5772: 54
48 Hahl to RKA 2.3.1908. RKA 5774: 3-7
49 Wick quarterly report 1.1.-31.3.1913, RKA 5772: 223
50 Wick quarterly report, 1.1.-31.3.1909, RKA 3774: 62

together with instructions on ways of ensuring clean water.[54] New books on preventive health measures or regaining and maintaining health in the tropics, superseding all such handbooks written before 1900, were also recommended.[55] Health checks and regulations applied to government employees only, and plantation company staff, missionaries and settlers continued to arrive without preliminary medical checks, a practice much deplored by doctors.

Baining Settlers

One group of people who took their chances were a few German families from Queensland who were persuaded to move to New Guinea by way of experiment. Keen to establish the extent to which Europeans could become acclimatised, and as a way of finding out whether permanent European settlement and small-scale farming was in fact possible, Governor Hahl devised a scheme to settle German farmers in the Gazelle Peninsula. The location for this experiment was the Baining Mountains, the western region of the Peninsula. Within reasonable reach of a harbour, the land was deemed suitable for small farmholdings and, at an altitude of 250 to 350 meters, it was thought to be free of anopheles. This assumption quickly proved false when the settlers began to suffer severely from malaria. Combined with other health problems, two men died within weeks of arrival. No questions had been asked about the state of health of the settlers; had they undergone a medical examination before going to New Guinea, four families would probably have been prevented from leaving Queensland. Two of the heads of families were over the age of fifty, one with a serious heart complaint, the other in poor health in general; another man also had a heart disorder, and one suffered from a chronic stomach disorder.[56] Given their state of health, some of the people were unlikely subjects for such an experiment.

As part of the financial support for the fledgling settlements, and perhaps also by way of compensation, the government provided free medical services and free hospital accommodation for the Baining settlers. One problem was transport to and from Herbertshöhe: people could not always get to a doctor

51   Wick quarterly report 1.4.-30.6.1913, RKA 5772: 252
52   Wick quarterly report 1.4.-30.6.1909, RKA 5771: 128
53   Wick quarterly report 1.1.-31.3.1913, RKA 5772: 223
54   *DKB* 13 (1902): 475-81
55   Recommended were among others C. Mense, *Tropische Gesundheitslehre und Heilkunde*, 1902; and F. Plehn, *Tropenhygiene: ärztliche Ratschläge für Kolonialbeamte, Offiziere, Missionare, Expeditionsführer, Pflanzer und Faktoristen*, 1902. Later also A. Plehn, *Kurzgefasste Vorschriften zur Verhütung und Behandlung tropischer Krankheiten*. 1906, Jena: Fischer. Also

in good time or, once they were at the hospital in Herbertshöhe, could not return home immediately so that for many a stay at the hospital at Herbertshöhe, and later in Rabaul, became a holiday. The alternative, a doctor's visit to the settlement, although it involved a two-day trip, was not uncommon.[57]

Tuberculosis

While malaria remained the overriding health problem, a number of other diseases gave rise for concern. Foremost were tuberculosis and sexually transmitted diseases.

In his article on tuberculosis in New Guinea, Wigley has suggested that Baroness von Schleinitz, the wife of the first German administrator, died of tuberculosis.[58] The Schleinitzes arrived in June 1886 and Frau von Schleinitz died on 18 January 1887, officially from diphtheria.[59] This was also the first reported death among the Europeans in the Kaiser-Wilhelmsland district. Wigley's argument that a euphemism was used to veil the true condition of the patient is plausible. Whether it was diphtheria or tuberculosis, it seems ironic that the first European death among the new settlers was from an introduced disease, not from malaria. It is also significant that tuberculosis, which was to have devastating effects on the native population, is suspected in this first European death. The first reported death from tuberculosis among the Germans was that of Jordan, the government secretary. He died in Surabaya on 17 February 1890, a few days after leaving Finschhafen to return to Germany.[60] He had spent three years at Finschhafen, but it is not known whether he was infected when he arrived. Over the next twenty-four years, numerous Europeans were infected, and a number died throughout the colony. Among those suffering from tuberculosis were missionaries and settlers, so that infection was possible wherever colonists had settled. Together with South Sea Islanders and Asians who brought tuberculosis with them, there were many possible infected contacts and New Guineans could not avoid tuberculosis.[61]

highly recommended "for English speakers", was Ronald Ross's *Malarial Fever, its Cause, Prevention and Treatment.*

56   MB 1905/6: 269-70

57   G255/737

58   S.C. Wigley, 'Tuberculosis and New Guinea', in B.G. Burton-Bradley, ed. *A History of Medicine in Papua New Guinea*, 179

Medical reports for German New Guinea list a total of nineteen Europeans who died of tuberculosis or suffered from tuberculosis when death occurred for another reason: fifteen in the Bismarck Archipelago administrative area, and four in Kaiser-Wilhelmsland.

In the Bismarck Archipelago, four victims belonged to the Sacred Heart Mission, two were traders, three planters[62]. Five persons were not identified by occupation[63]. Of the missionaries, one nun died in 1901 after six years in the Bismarck Archipelago, the other died in 1906 at Vunapope after three and a half years in the colony. Father Gouthéraud died at St. Otto in the Baining mountains, having spent nineteen years in the Bismarck Archipelago. Brother Dannbauer died after eighteen months in the colony of meningitis, with a note by Dr Wendland that it was most likely tuberculosis based. One of the traders died in 1899, the other, a "half Samoan", had lived on the island of Nugarea, and had spent his whole life in the colony. One unidentified man who died of tuberculosis on Matupi had been in the colony for ten years; his pulmonary tuberculosis had first been positively diagnosed in 1903. The seaman who died of pulmonary tuberculosis had been on the survey ship *Möwe*. The other settler treated during 1903 was a planter, who had been in the country for several years and died in 1905.

Of the four tuberculosis deaths in Kaiser-Wilhelmsland, one was that of a government employee, one of a Catholic missionary who died at Tumleo, the third of a nun who died at Eitape. The fourth was that of a planter who died at Aroka after having lived in the colony for ten years.

To complete the picture we should look at patients listed in medical reports as suffering from tuberculosis. As early as 1903 Wendland pointed out that tuberculosis was increasing among natives and labourers and therefore, in the interest of the individuals themselves and of the local population, sufferers or suspects, should not be sent to New Guinea.[64] Wendland voiced his concern in strong terms, pointing out that the practice of the Catholic Mission of sending people suffering or suspected of suffering from tuberculosis to the milder climate of the tropics was a contributing factor in the increase of tuberculosis in the indigenous population. He was in no doubt that the close contact between missionaries and unexposed people gave rise to a very high risk of infection. However, the Colonial Department edited Wendland's con-

59   *NKWL* 1887: 136. In his memoirs Schellong described Mrs Schleinitz as suffering from "septic diphtheria", of which she died within a few days. Schellong, *Alte Dokumente* 109. If and to what extent malaria was a factor must remain speculative.

60   *NKWL* 1890: 8

demnation into a very general statement as it was feared that "the powerful influence of the Sacred Heart Mission could lead to much unpleasantness for Dr Wendland."[65]

There were a number of sufferers at the Catholic mission: one priest was diagnosed from the time of his arrival and Wendland suspected that other missionaries were suffering also. How much heed was taken of his warning is impossible to say, but it does not appear that infected mission staff were repatriated immediately, as in 1906 a nun who died of tuberculosis at Vunapope had been ill there for three years and one priest suffering from tuberculosis left the colony in 1907. Brother Dannbauer, who died in 1907, had been at Vunapope for eighteen months. Another nun was sent home from Vunapope in 1910 because of tuberculosis.[66]

The pattern among Catholic missionaries was repeated in Kaiser-Wilhelmsland at the Divine Word Mission. In 1908 a priest died of tuberculosis and in 1910 a nun died at Eitape. A nun from Kaiser-Wilhelmsland left New Guinea in 1909 because of tuberculosis.

Dr Hoffmann, at Friedrich-Wilhelmshafen, repeated the warning about sending sufferers or suspects to New Guinea in 1908. "Inevitable malaria" only made the tuberculosis problem worse; in addition a sufferer posed a definite threat to a native population where the incidence was "not yet" widespread.[67] By 1909 doctors' warnings became more urgent; as the number of cases among the native population was increasing annually, "it needed serious attention because of a threat to public health".[68] By 1910 Hoffmann's comment was seen as applicable to the whole colony:

> Tuberculosis is a serious threat to natives. A lack of old healed lesions noticed during autopsies, as would be seen in a large percentage of Europeans, proves that tuberculosis has been introduced into the colony only in recent times, most likely through Europeans. Every doctor here knows of cases where Europeans with highly advanced tuberculosis were in close contact with natives—be they missionaries, traders or planters—and disregarded precautionary measures of any sort and ensured the spread of the disease.[69]

---

61 Wigley 167 ff
62 One of whom was Richard Parkinson who died aged 65, following an operation for a tubercular hip joint, tuberculosis having been diagnosed 18 months before his death.
63 Indications are that an 18 year old man was a son of Richard Parkinson.
64 MB 1903/04:189-90

Doctors were unequivocal that Europeans had introduced tuberculosis and were still doing so. Repatriation was one way of dealing with patients, yet there is evidence of only one compulsory case. Dr Schlafke, the company medical officer in Friedrich-Wilhelmshafen, was sent back to Germany by Professor Koch in January 1900, eleven months after his arrival, following a tuberculosis diagnosis. Schlafke died within a year, presumably from tuberculosis.[70] Just how much pressure was exerted by a doctor to encourage an infected person to leave the colony is difficult to judge. In 1907 one man left on medical advice because of tuberculosis, and another did so in 1908. In Kaiser-Wilhelmsland the wife of a company employee left in 1909, "as the climate in German New Guinea was not congenial for tuberculosis sufferers"[71] and two men from Friedrich-Wilhelmshafen left the country because of tuberculosis in 1910.[72]

Venereal Disease

Venereal infection was intractable. As in the battle against malaria, so in that against venereal disease: human nature played an important part in its management and cure. Of the various types of infection gonorrhoea was the most prevalent. Of 137 cases of venereal infection treated at Rabaul from 1903 to 1911, ninety-six were gonorrhoea, including complications, twenty-eight were syphilis, six venereal condyloma and seven venereal buboes. Particularly in the cases of syphilis, the patients usually belonged to ships' crews and had brought the infection with them. The aim of the doctors was to contain the spread of disease, and while they seem to have been successful in that none of the Japanese prostitutes at the Rabaul brothels had to be treated for syphilis, there were large numbers of gonorrhoea treatments. Nevertheless, venereal disease seemed to be on the increase, and brothels were seen as a threat to the European population. Doctors tried two countermeasures. The first was an increase in medical examination of prostitutes from weekly to bi-weekly. The second was to draw the attention of customers to the possible danger to health and to recommend "suitable precautions". Unfortunately, no increase in the sale of "suitable items" was noticed in the pharmacy at Rabaul.[73]

---

65 Internal memoranda AA Steubel/Rose, 29.11. and 1.12.1904. RKA 5769: 96-7
66 MB 1906/07: 202-3; MB 1910/11: 641
67 MB 1908/9: 385, 391
68 MB 1909/10: 486
69 MB 1911/12: 497-8

Originally, a brothel had been set up quietly as a public health measure. Governor Hahl and Bishop Couppé agreed that in the interest of public health it was judicious to allow a brothel on Matupi. The increasing number of Europeans "of low social rank" who came to Matupi with naval and other vessels, together with the numerous Chinese who lived there, made it impossible to suppress prostitution. From a moral and a health point of view the involvement of native women in prostitution had to be avoided. Neither the mission nor the government were keen to have uncontrolled prostitution. Hahl's solution was ingenious, one possibly suggested by widespread Japanese prostitution in parts of South Asia, and also in northern Australia from the 1880s to early this century.[74] By introducing another group of women into the colony as prostitutes, local women were saved from depravity, which satisfied the Bishop. The government was satisfied also because it could dictate the terms under which these women were allowed entry and residence. If they created problems or refused regular medical examination, they could be expelled. On this basis, Hahl came to an understanding with the Chinese merchant Ah Tam: the government would not object to three Japanese prostitutes working at Ah Tam's hotel in Matupi provided they gave no cause for complaints of any sort and had regular medical examinations.[75] When the new capital was set up, Ah Tam moved this part of his business to Rabaul where it expanded quickly. By the end of 1913 there were between twenty and thirty Japanese prostitutes working there. During that year Dr Kersten treated 119 cases of gonorrhoea among natives, Chinese, and Japanese in addition to an unstated number of "unscrupulous Europeans". Medical control of prostitutes was carried out regularly, and infected women were treated.[76] However, there was no such control on the clientele and the result was a circular problem: examination and treatment for labourers under contract and domestic servants was compulsory, but not for men from other races. "Too many European men [were] gadding about with untreated gonorrhoea, even with syphilis, posing a constant danger for blacks and whites alike", according to Dr Runge.[77] Reinfection and cross-infection occurred despite regular testing and

70   RKA 5729: 36
71   MB 1909/10: 486
72   MB 1910/11: 680
73   Kopp, quarterly report 1.10.-31.12.1911, RKA 5772: 121
74   See for instance the section on Japanese prostitution in Susan Jane Hunt, *Spinifex and Hessian: Women's Lives in North-Western Australia 1869-1900* (Nedland:, UWA Press, 1986) 123 ff. Also D.C.S. Sisson, 'Karayuki-San: Japanese prostitution in Australia, 1887-1916', *Historical Studies* 17 (1976/77): 323-41, 474-88

treatment of prostitutes. Chinese men also posed a difficult problem, as they tended to seek medical help only at the point of death.[78] A new threat to public health had also arisen because native men had begun to visit the establishment despite strictest prohibition, and this in turn exposed local women to infection. By the end of 1914 it looked as if gonorrhoea had begun its "victory march"[79] despite valiant efforts by the authorities.

Hookworm and Other Problems

Intestinal parasites first appeared on the medical agenda when Professor Koch during his visit to New Guinea drew to the attention of doctors the prevalence of *anchylostomum duodenale* (hookworm).[80] Hookworm treatment with Thymol became routine in native hospitals if it was found that worm infestation was the cause of anaemia; it was a health problem restricted to natives and Chinese. Or so it seemed until 1912, when Dr Kopp decided to examine the children at the European school at Namanula. Twelve of the fifteen children were found to be worm infested. The three who were free of hookworm wore shoes at all times. Thymol treatment, and an insistence that white children wore shoes at all times, cured the problem temporarily,[81] but as a result of the hookworm infestation local residents began to agitate to have the government school for native children moved from Namanula to downtown Rabaul. These children were seen as a health threat: they suffered from malaria and were worm infested and both conditions could be spread easily to white children living in Namanula. The move of the native school was eventually planned for 1915.[82]

A doctor in New Guinea dealt with a wide range of routine problems. Innumerable surgical cases required minor operations. Quite large operations were also carried out, such as amputations. For such surgery it was usual to include a surgeon from a naval ship in the operating team. In the case of Richard Parkinson, for instance, the medical team consisted of the two resident doctors Born and Wick, and Dr Schütze from the survey vessel *Planet*.[83]

75   Hahl to AA 23.11.1904, RKA 2991:74-75

76   Kersten, 'Die Gonorrhöe im Bezirk Rabaul (Deutsch-Neuguinea)', *ASTH* 29 (1925), Beiheft 1: 180-3. Also his quarterly report 1.7.-30.9.1913, RKA 5772: 267

77   Runge, quarterly report 1.1.-31.3.1912, RKA 5772: 159 ff

78   Kersten, quarterly report 1.1.-31.3.1914, RKA 5773: 107 ff

79   Kersten, op. cit. 180

80   AR NGC 1899/1900: 21. It is notable that a hookworm eradication campaign began in Germany in 1903. See H.H. Scott, *A History of Tropical Medicine* (London, Edward Arnold & Co., 1939), vol. 2, 848

Doctors had to undertake some minor emergency dental work also but, as government employees were expected to have dental treatment during home leave, such work was not common. A clash between District Officer Boluminski in Kaewieng and the government about payment for dental work on government employees undertaken by a visiting dentist[84] led to a change in this regulation. In any case, the increased population required a properly qualified dentist. During his home leave in 1912 Dr Runge, government medical officer in Herbertshöhe, trained as a dentist, and two medical orderlies, Faulenbach in Rabaul and Lachmann in Kaewieng, trained as dental technicians, all at government expense.[85] Typically, treatment entitlement and associated cost were closely regulated by the government.[86]

Utopia in German New Guinea

Much to the vexation of doctors a tiny minority of colonists refused to submit to any medical authority—the 'Brothers of the Order of the Sun' (*Sonnenbrüder*).[87] The founder of the Order and self-styled leader was Augustus Engelhardt, who decided to set up his utopia in New Guinea. He bought Kabakon Island (in the Duke of York group) from Forsayth & Company in 1903 to build there "a future free from worries" for himself and his disciples. His gospel was the power of the sun and the coconut. According to Engelhardt, coconuts were the complete and only food required and the panacea for all illness. Clothing was anathema also—to fully enjoy the benefits of the sun the whole body had to be exposed, so the "cocovores" went around naked, and put on a loin cloth only when visitors came to the island. Engelhardt persuaded a few 'brothers' to join him and become "cocovores" on Kabakon. Over a period of years a number of disciples arrived. Needless to say, malaria caught up with them very quickly. Four died within months of arrival, and two returned to Germany. Engelhardt managed to acquire immunity against malaria and was still on Kabakon when war broke out; apart

81   RKA 5772: 186
82   Draft Budget 1915: 58, G255/754
83   RKA 5771: 145-7; RKA 5772: 134
84   G255/644: 131ff. A Dr Moon visited the colony and carried out dental work on a number of people, among them government employees
85   RKA 5731: 133
86   A circular to all government stations set the grounds on which a government employee was entitled to free dental treatment as well as costs to private persons. RKA 5731: 132 ff. Regulation also published in *Amtsblatt* 1914: 169-70

from growing coconuts, he had established a business supplying New Guinea plants and plant extracts to a German pharmacist for the production of medications.

Dr Wendland quickly diagnosed Engelhardt as "paranoid" and was most distressed that ideas of this nature should be propagated in Germany, encouraging others in the foolhardy enterprise.[88] The government took a dim view of the prospects of the "apostles of the coconut". Their overt rejection of professional advice and medical authority raised concerns about possible costs to the public purse, and each 'brother' was required to pay a bond of 800 Mark in case hospitalisation or repatriation became necessary. There is no evidence to suggest that any other settler was required to lodge such a bond, but they subscribed to accepted doctrines of health.

Self-Help

Another concern of the administration and doctors was the range of patent medicines of foreign origin that were used by settlers.[89] The unsupervised and liberal use of "English panaceas" such as Elliman's Embrocation, Bronchitis Cure and Painkiller, the latter two mixtures containing morphine and chloroform, were regarded with great misgivings by doctors.[90] However, as many settlers lived nowhere near a doctor or a hospital dispensary, self-reliance was necessary for treating both themselves and their labourers. Large plantation owners and missions kept their own dispensaries and imported bulk pharmaceutical supplies direct from Germany or Australia, keeping purchases from the hospital dispensary to a minimum. Small settlers bought their pharmaceuticals either from a plantation dispensary or from the hospital dispensary. In this way there was a considerable traffic in pharmaceutical supplies without medical supervision, and prices varied a great deal throughout the colony. Therefore, in order to encourage small settlers to purchase supplies from a hospital dispensary, prices were fixed by the government at the lowest level possible while at the same time giving doctors discretion in selling goods at cost price to indigent settlers or natives.[91] This pricing arrangement also gave doctors the opportunity to monitor the use of medications to a certain extent.

---

87   I am indebted to Dr Berenwenger for material which enabled me to piece together the story of the "Order of the Sun". See also Hermann J. Hiery, 'Germans, Pacific Islanders and Sexuality' in Hermann J. Hiery and John M. MacKenzie, eds., *European Impact and Pacific Influence* (London/New York: Tauris Academic Studies, 1997) 303

88   MB 1905/06:259-61; MB 1906/07: 215

New Guinea was not the only colony with problems in the supply of medications and, to bring the rules for pharmacies and the supply of medications into line with those in Germany, new regulations came into force throughout the colonies on 1 May 1911.[92] For New Guinea this meant in practice that, apart from the hospital dispensaries in Rabaul, Herbertshöhe, Kaewieng, Namatanai, Kieta and Friedrich-Wilhelmshafen which were under the supervision of a government doctor, and the dispensary in the hospital of the New Guinea Company in Friedrich-Wilhelmshafen as long as it was under the supervision of a government doctor, there were a number of licensed *Hausapotheken,* 'domestic dispensaries'. The main 'domestic' licensees were mission stations and the major plantation companies,[93] all subject to the supervision of a government medical officer or other person authorised by the government. The first private pharmacy was opened in Rabaul on 15 January 1912 by Mr. E. Paur, a qualified pharmacist.[94]

Despite tight regulations, the use of patent medicines from sources other than pharmacies continued.[95] To the medical concern of doctors about the widespread use and abuse of patent medicines was added that of the pharmacist, whose business interests were directly affected. The issue was not resolved before the outbreak of the war.

Nutrition

Theories current in Germany on the acclimatisation of Europeans in the tropics, and on helping to maintain their health, emphasised good nutrition. Schellong's articles seemed to have been seminal on the subject. Apart from suitable housing, appropriate to a tropical climate, plenty of water tanks, and "a certain heroism" needed for the regular intake of quinine, he placed great

89 Hahl to RKA 6.12.1907 in RKA 5820: 4-5
90 MB 1910/11: 660
91 Circular to district officers/doctors 20.8.1907 re pricing of medications. RKA 5820: 6
92 Verordnung des Reichskanzlers betr. die Einrichtung und den Betrieb von Apotheken in den deutschen Schutzgebieten mit Ausnahme von Deutsch-Südwest Afrika, 12 January 1911 (*DKB* 22(1911): 42-44
93 The Methodist Mission stations in Ula, Kabakada, Vatnabara, Namatanai, Omo and Raluana; the Catholic Mission station at Vunapope; the NGC stations in Peterhafen, Massava, Herbertshöhe, Towakundum, Wunawutang, Wangaramut; the Forsayth Company plantation hospital at Bitalobo; Hernsheim & Co. in Matupi, Makada, Portland Islands and Manus; J.M. Rondahl at Kulon, Makurapau and Kabakaul; the Neuendettelsau Mission stations at Finschhafen and Deinzer-Höhe; the Rhenish Mission at Bogadjim; the SVD Mission station at St Michael (Eitape district); H.R. Wahlen Co. on its stations in the Ninigo and Hermit Groups and Manus. *Amtsblatt* 1914: 94-5

importance on plentiful fresh food.[96] However, a diet similar to the one to which people were accustomed at home was difficult to achieve in Kaiser-Wilhelmsland. The New Guinea Company alluded to problems: in Finschhafen "under the given conditions general requirements of hygiene could not be met in all respects."[97] This was confirmed by Knappe, the German vice-consul in Apia, who spent the months of July and August 1886 there. His report to Chancellor Bismarck[98] described accommodation in the so called Swedish houses as "cells" measuring 6' x 8', equipped with a narrow bed, and the rest of the furniture made from wooden boxes. Food supply was inadequate in that for several weeks the diet consisted in the main of salt meat and bread made from mouldy flour. The canteen had prices worked out in Berlin, but not much was on offer. The anxiously awaited company supply steamer *Ottilie* arrived without stores, so that the *Samoa* had to be dispatched to Mioko and Matupi to obtain urgently need-ed supplies from the trading firms DHPG and Hernsheim. The company was less than sympathetic to complaints. Hansemann refuted allegations and argued that, quite apart from the fact that Knappe's report was one-sided, if food stores had deteriorated it was because of incorrect storage, hence clear-ly the fault of the personnel at Finschhafen. As for accommodation, larger houses were on the way. In any case, prospective employees had been warned that they were going to undertake pioneering work and some hard-ships had to be expected.[99]

There is enough evidence to show that the logistics of food supplies remained a problem for some years. Kindt, the manager of Erima station, complained that he was unable to get adequate food supplies for himself and his family from the Finschhafen store, contrary to assurances given to him in Berlin. They had to subsist on rice, and he claimed that because of poor nutri-tion they were unable to recover from severe malaria attacks. His youngest child aged fifteen months had died because the company was not able to supply milk when his supplies of tinned milk ran out. He was only able to replenish his stores when he went to Mioko and Matupi himself in April 1891.[100] Kindt's complaints were dismissed by the company on the grounds that he

---

94   *Amtsblatt* 1912: 4
95   RKA 5820: 76 ff
96   O. Schellong, 'Tropenhygienische Betrachtungen', *DKZ* 5 (1888): 341-3; 363-4; 368-71. Others to take up the topic were, for instance, C.E. Ranke, *Ueber die Einwirkung des Tropenklimas auf die Ernährung des Menschen.* (Berlin, 1900).
97   *NKWL* 1886: 84
98   RKA 2977: 11-31

had been warned not to take his family with him and the death of his child was due to illness, not lack of food—which was probably true. In any case, Kindt's complaint was to be viewed with some reservations; he no doubt had a grudge against the company as he had been sacked because of ill-treatment of his labourers, and he was also known for ill-treating his wife and family.[101]

The commander of the naval cruiser *Leipzig* could not be dismissed so easily. When the cruiser called at Finschhafen, food was short because of lack of shipping, and it had to help out with urgently needed flour, sugar and other staples.[102]. Sister Hertzer also confirmed problems with food supplies when she noted that "There is virtually nothing left to eat, and nobody feels like eating the few things that are still available here. My hens are laying only every second day; we are in a bad way here".[103]

In order to combat chronic anaemia, doctors advised plentiful fresh meat. This led to the importation of cattle. Again, there were problems: cattle imported from Australia in April 1885 had done well when they were checked a few months later. The only problem was that the beasts had grown wild and it was impossible to catch and bring them to Finschhafen.[104] Cattle breeding turned out to be very troublesome and suffered setbacks. Australian cattle perished on board ship before reaching Friedrich-Wilhelmshafen, and from the next shipment three quarters of the animals died from an unidentified disease shortly after arrival in Friedrich-Wilhelmshafen.[105] Poultry in Hatzfeldhafen suffered likewise from some unknown disease and died.[106] The stock was gradually built up and by 1896 there were enough cattle for slaughtering every third day.[107] In the Bismarck Archipelago Imperial Commissioner Rose found that cattle breeding to supply fresh meat and milk to Europeans was expensive and that it would be better for individuals to trade for fish and meat with natives, and keep a few cows on a plantation for the supply of milk.[108]

Many attempts were made to improve the diet by planting European vegetables. While there were reasonable results initially in Finschhafen and in Hatzfeldhafen,[109] Schellong noted that vegetables did not grow and imported potatoes did not keep for long after arrival. Settlers had to rely on a

99   Hansemann to Bismarck, RKA 2977: 48 ff

100 Kindt to Chancellor Caprivi, RKA 2410: 26-32

101 Hansemann to Caprivi, RKA 2410: 42 ff

102 Report by commander Valois of cruiser squadron, 3.9.1890, RKA 2979: 102

103 Hertzer diary, 11 December 1891

104 *NKWL* 1886: 66

105 *NKWL* 1893: 20-21

106 *NKWL* 1886: 83

107 *NKWL* 1896: 14

monotonous diet of tinned food for months at a time.[110] In 1889 there were reports of crop failures because of leaf-eating insects and drought.[111] The potato crop in Constantinhafen was attacked by enormous masses of caterpillars. It was not until 1896 that Stephansort station reported a satisfactory supply of milk, vegetables and fruit.[112]

Much to the concern of doctors, as late as 1912 settlers still depended on a large amount of tinned food from Germany or Australia. Regular shipping ensured that there were no food shortages, but doctors on all stations except Rabaul pointed out that the quantity of tinned food was too large in relation to fresh food. Unless settlers kept poultry and planted a vegetable garden, fresh meat and vegetables were still difficult to obtain. Only married men with families who planned for a long term future in the colony were likely to make that effort. "A certain indolence" prevented many from doing likewise and they relied entirely on tins. Hunting large pigeons, which had provided some fresh meat in the early days, brought few results around Friedrich-Wilhelmshafen, Herbertshöhe and Kaewieng. Everywhere natives were loath to sell fresh food such as fish or pigs to settlers.

In Rabaul food supply was better as Chinese market gardeners had vegetables for sale. Refrigerated ships brought fresh meat, vegetables and fruit regularly from Australia and, when ice became available with the establishment of an ice works in 1911, supplies could be stored. Nevertheless, although food supplies were excellent, they were dear.[113]

Together with imported drink and household goods, the cost of living was very high anywhere in the colony. This high cost—a source of constant complaints—was probably manageable by government and company employees with a regular income and colonial allowances, but it may have been different for small settlers. The case of the wife of a Baining settler suffering from malaria and malnutrition[114] suggests that not all settlers were in a position to grow sufficient food for themselves, nor able to buy adequate supplies of the expensive imported food.

108 Rose report 1.1.1891-30.6.1892, RKA 6512: 104
109 *NKWL* 1886: 65; 1888: 150-1
110 O. Schellong, 'Die Neu-Guinea Malaria einst und jetzt', *ASTH* 5 (1901): 307
111 *NKWL* 1889: 23
112 *NKWL* 1896: 14
113 MB 1911/12: 486-88

INFRASTRUCTURE

Hospitals and Nursing

The need for hospitals became obvious very early. From the very beginning a racial distinction was made and separate hospitals were built for Europeans (*Europäerkrankenhaus*) and for labourers (*Eingeborenenkrankenhaus*). Initially the demand for a European hospital came from doctors so that nursing care could be given by professional staff. Most New Guinea Company employees in the colony were single men, without wifely care during illness, and provision had to be made for them. This argument was reversed after the turn of the century when it was pointed out that, because women and children were in the colony, a hospital was needed. A hospital also became a focus for the settler communities. Women in the widely dispersed settlements found a temporary refuge from isolation and loneliness; there they obtained not only medical attention but also the support and company of other European women. When the new European hospital for Rabaul was planned, the Rabaul branch of the *Kolonialer Frauenbund* [the Colonial Women's League][115] agitated for a women's wing, to accommodate women already in the colony and as an encouragement to others to immigrate.[116] It also supported the building of a hospital in Kaewieng, with special facilities for women.[117] The league's committee was involved in decorating the new Rabaul government hospital, especially the women's ward.[118]

Dr Schellong, soon after his arrival, was the first doctor to agitate for a European hospital. Primitive and cramped accommodation was very uncomfortable for patients and doctor. Of greater importance was the need for basic nursing care, in a situation made worse by the utter lack of fellow-feeling among colonists; although fever was a daily occurrence, no one felt obliged to look after a sick neighbour.[119] When the hospital for Europeans was final-

114 MB 1911/12: 513
115 The Colonial Women's League was founded in 1907 and was closely affiliated with the German Colonial Society. The aim of the league was to promote the emigration of German women to the colonies and to support them there, "for each German woman who goes to a colony lifts its cultural level". The founding committee was made up mostly of wives of officers serving in the Colonial Troops (*DKZ* 22 (1905): 122; 24 (1907): 137; 144). A branch was founded in Rabaul in 1909 which virtually all government employees and settlers and their wives joined (*Amtsblatt* 15.10.1909, supplement 3-4).
116 *Amtsblatt* 1911: 118-9, appeal by Mrs. Hahl, president of the Women's League in Rabaul
117 *Amtsblatt* 1914: 109,
118 *Amtsblatt* 1914: 213

ly ready there remained the problem of nursing, for, as Schellong pointed out, "this tiring and devoted task is not within a man's province".[120] As an interim measure, Schellong suggested that personal servants be employed, preferably Melanesian boys, who could be trained readily.[121] In practice it was more likely that a single man would set up house with a woman recruited as a labourer.

The first assistant for Schellong had arrived in June 1886—a young man by the name of Martin, a surgical instrument maker by trade; but he had resigned by the time the hospital opened. Together with the boy Tom from Mioko he had taken care of the sick—Europeans and labourers—as well as could be managed, but his prospects looked better in Australia. The second assistant was a locksmith (*Schlosser*), willing but clumsy. He died seven months later of malaria, in October 1887.[122] By that time the first qualified medical orderly had arrived, Carl Boschat, who had been trained at the Charité Hospital in Berlin.[123] For Boschat it was the beginning of a thirteen years' association with the colony.[124]

The first nurses finally arrived in June 1891, Sisters Auguste Hertzer and Hedwig Saul, who took charge of the European hospital at Stephansort.[125] They were employed by the German Women's Association for Nursing in the Colonies.[126] Another two nurses followed in June 1892—Sisters Knigge and Kubanke. They had trained at the Augusta-Hospital in

119 Schellong, 'Neu-Guinea Malaria' 311

120 Schellong, *Alte Dokumente* 102-3

121 Schellong, *Alte Dokumente* 103. Administrator von Schleinitz had taken the precaution of bringing his own personal staff.

122 Schellong, *Alte Dokumente* 85, 100, 113, 117; 173

123 Schellong, *Alte Dokumente* 149. The Charité Hospital was a very well known 4000-bed state hospital, closely associated with the name of Virchow and later Koch. See T.D. Brock, *Robert Koch, a Life in Medicine and Bacteriology* (Madison: Science Tech Publishers, 1986) 14

124 Boschat died in FWH on 10 March 1900 of influenza and his wife died a few days later (AR NGC 1899/1900:17; 'Monumental inscriptions in the German Cemetery, Madang', *Progenitor* 6 (1987): 13

125 *NKWL* 1891: 25. By that time Finschhafen had been abandoned as a result of the many deaths that occurred there from the beginning of January to mid-March 1891 and new headquarters were set up at Stephansort, near Friedrich-Wilhelmshafen.

126 The *Deutscher Frauenverein für Krankenpflege in den Kolonien* was founded in 1888, sponsored by the *Deutsch-nationaler Frauenbund* (Patriotic Women's League). Its main objective was the co-ordination of nursing in the colonies and the training of nurses to work in hospitals for Europeans in the colonies and also military hospitals in time of war. The association supported nurses during their 18 months training—from mid-1890s on in the *Neues Allgemeines Krankenhaus* in Hamburg-Eppendorf. After the turn of the century a course at the Institute for Ships' and Tropical Diseases in Hamburg was added to the nurses' train-

Berlin.[127] In the following year Sister Anna Meyer came to Friedrich-Wilhelmshafen to replace Kubanke, who had to leave because of ill health.[128] The New Guinea Company provided board and lodging for the nurses and a small amount of pocket money.

The importance of personal nursing was much emphasised by Dempwolff, who was sure that "careful nursing in hospital, an encouraging word at the right moment, good food and good drink had saved many lives. A few men were lucky enough to have a loving wife taking care of them during illness. Most others owed a great debt of gratitude to the tireless efforts of the Red Cross nurse."[129]

Apart from careful nursing, Dempwolff's prescription was quinine and hydrotherapy. In extreme cases the quantity of quinine given ranged from 0.5 to 1.5 grams every six hours until the fever subsided completely. There was hardly a case for which he did not prescribe hydrotherapy: cold compresses, enemas, showers, baths at an exact temperature and steam baths. When the patient was better, he was given various forms of iron to counter anaemia.[130] It is not surprising that he praised the devoted work of nurses; the intensive care of patients was entirely in their hands. There was little acknowledgement of their work later, although they were essential if a European hospital was to serve its purpose. Despite the fact that there was a nearly continuous presence of nurses in New Guinea, very few records attest to their work or even to their existence. With the exception of Auguste Hertzer we have nothing but a name, others remain anonymous. (See Appendix III for a list of the nurses who worked in New Guinea as far as can be established.)

From the outset, as part of their duties nurses also took charge of all domestic

ing. The association paid for the trip to and from a colony, a large part of nurses' salaries, and fitted them out before departure; it also equipped hospitals and nurses' quarters. It became affiliated with the Red Cross in 1909, under the name *Deutscher Frauenverein vom Roten Kreuz für die Kolonien*. Increasingly nurses trained also as midwives for 6 or 9 months at the Charité in Berlin or the women's clinics of university hospitals before leaving for the colonies. Most of the nurses went to work in the African colonies. The association enjoyed the patronage of the Empress. Although the association received funding from the *Wohlfahrtslotterie* [Welfare Lottery], it continued fund raising activities. With the Empress as patroness of the association, such functions were highly prestigious occasions. *DKZ* 5 (1888): 316-17; 13 (1896):433-34; 14 (1897): 165. Kimmle, ed., *Das Deutsche Rote Kreuz* (Berlin: Boll & Pickardt, 1910) vol. 2: 665-703

127 *NKWL* 1892: 39

128 *DKB* 5 (1894): 377

129 Dempwolff, 'Aerztliche Erfahrungen' 152; 278. Governor Hahl was among them when he suffered malaria and dysentery and later severe attacks of blackwater fever. Hahl, *Governor in New Guinea*, translated and edited by P. Sack & D. Clark (Canberra, ANU Press, 1980) 93

130 Dempwolff, 'Aerztliche Erfahrungen' 151

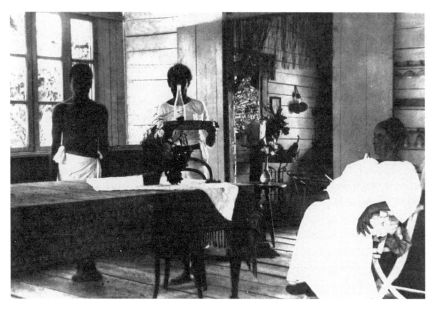

Sister Auguste Hertzer at home

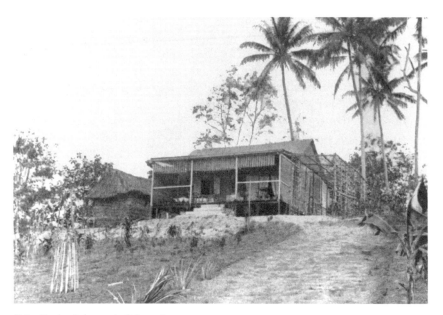

Sister Hertzer's house in Palaupai

arrangements necessary to run a hospital, including the supervision of kitchens and kitchen gardens. The ratio of nurses to patients was high, as Jackman suggests, if it is considered that they were looking after Europeans only.[131] There is no doubt that much more time was devoted to a patient in European hospitals than in the native hospitals. Nevertheless, it needs to be remembered that nurses, and for that matter medical orderlies—whose province was native hospitals— suffered from malaria also. Like all other people, intermittently they were unfit to work.[132]

The European hospital in Finschhafen was ready on 16 December 1887,[133] two years after the arrival of the first settlers. It was a prefabricated wooden building, consisting of one large room with seven beds and two small single rooms for seriously ill patients.[134] When Finschhafen was evacuated in 1891, the hospital was dismantled and rebuilt on Beliao Peninsula, together with a house to accommodate the doctor and the nursing sisters. The "old and dilapidated" hospital was no longer usable by 1895, and the former residence of Landeshauptmann Schmiele was converted to accommodate the doctor and double as a European hospital. By this time the main operations of the company had been moved to Stephansort and there were only about seven Europeans at Friedrich-Wilhelmshafen. The main hospital was now set up at Stephansort with Sister Hertzer in charge,[135] and it in turn was abandoned when operations ceased. Following this reorganisation, the company built a new five-bed hospital in 1901 in Friedrich-Wilhelmshafen on Beliao Peninsula and also a doctor's residence. The hospital was built of wood, standing on cement posts, and covered by a corrugated iron roof. It consisted of two large rooms and four smaller rooms. One of the large rooms at the front was the nurse's living quarters. The other large room was equipped to accommodate two patients, and three of the smaller rooms accommodated one patient each; thus five patients could be accommodated "comfortably". The fourth smaller room was used as a "bandaging room". Rainwater was stored in large tanks and there was also a well on the island. An enthusiastic

---

131 Jackman, 'Malaria in German New Guinea' 129
132 Hedwig Saul suffered from repeated and severe fever (*NKWL* 1892: 38). Emma Kubanke "managed to fulfil her contract in New Guinea despite severe illness" and Nurse Knigge had to leave New Guinea after a year despite a convalescent trip to Singapore (*DKB* 5 (1894): 377). In 1894 when Sister Hertzer was in sole charge of the European hospital in Friedrich-Wilhelmshafen, she had to spend some weeks in Java for recuperation following severe malaria *DKB* 5 (1894): 377.
133 *NKWL* 1888: 58. See Appendix VIII for list of hospitals 1887-1915
134 Schellong, *Alte Dokumente* 185
135 *NKWL* 1896: 9

gardener among the company employees set up and maintained a vegetable garden to supply the hospital and staff, so that tinned food could be kept to a minimum. After his death nobody bothered to continue the work and the garden fell into disuse. Sanitary installations were minimal, and Hoffmann recommended that sewerage pipes be laid to carry sewage directly into the sea.[136] By 1907 the hospital "no longer corresponded to modern needs of tropical hospitals" in that the rooms were too low and too small. The wood was infested with white ants; all in all the old hospital had to be replaced.[137] However, it took years before a new government hospital was funded. As usual, allocation of funds was a balancing act, and while there was some sort of hospital for the few Europeans living in Kaiser-Wilhelmsland, Hahl was not keen to give high priority to a new hospital in Friedrich-Wilhelmshafen. Under the contract between the Reich and the New Guinea Company, the old hospital remained the property and responsibility of the company. "Some necessary repairs" were carried out in 1908[138] and again in 1911. Thus repaired, but still quite ramshackle, the hospital had to suffice until a government hospital was built.[139] Despite the recognition of the urgent need for a new hospital, with the governor pointing out that "care must be taken of Friedrich-Wilhelmshafen before a European hospital can be built anywhere in the colony,[140] it only became part of the budget plan for 1915.[141] As will be seen later, pressure from Kaewieng residents for a new hospital was such that they were given precedence.

On the Gazelle Peninsula, a hospital for Europeans was included in the initial planning for the transfer of the government from Friedrich-Wilhelmshafen to Herbertshöhe. The temporary house for the governor built in 1899 could readily be converted for use as a hospital for Europeans.[142] Meantime the doctor treated all patients at their homes. For people outside Herbertshöhe, it was usually possible to lodge with friends, or in the local hotel. Others preferred to go to Sydney. It was also possible for Europeans to go to the polyclinic which had been set up for labourers and natives, which, according to Wendland, was perfectly adequate provided the European patient was "not spoilt".[143] The need for a hospital for Europeans was advo-

136 Annual Report 1901/02: 232.; MB 1903/04: 208; 1907/08: 444
137 MB 1907/08: 445
138 MB 1908/09: 385
139 MB 1911/12: 481
140 Hahl to Kaewieng District Office 12.7.1913. G255/892: 1a
141 Draft budget 1915, G255/754
142 AR 1899-1900: 199
143 Denkschrift, Anlage Aktenstück 54, *Stenographische Berichte der Verhandlungen des Reichstags,* 1903/04 (11. Legislatur-periode, 2. Session) 1. Anlageband, 397

cated by Wendland, but he was emphatic that a hospital for labourers and natives was far more urgent.[144] How much agitation occurred on the part of newcomers is impossible to say.

The conversion of the old governor's residence to a European hospital was completed in February 1904. The hospital consisted of five rooms and accommodated four to six patients.[145] The building was Berlin's contribution to tropical architecture and had peculiar design features: it lacked any windows; in their place were twenty-seven wooden doors in the style of French windows. The lower section of the door was solid wood; the upper section had shutter-like slats in place of glass panes. As Wendland wryly commented, this construction provided plenty of ventilation, but not much light, and was particularly unfortunate if surgery had to be carried out; there was either plenty of light and dust, or no light and not quite so much dust.[146] The hospital was at times completely occupied, particularly when ships' crews needed hospitalisation. The tradition of sending patients to Brisbane or Sydney was also upheld, particularly when a long recuperation was expected and the patient could afford the trip.[147]

It was soon necessary to enlarge the hospital to seven beds. A separate house was also built for the nurse. She was on duty day and night, and patients had an electric bell at their bed with which they could summon her from her house.[148] Nevertheless, their work at Herbertshöhe was not as hard as it had been in Friedrich-Wilhelmshafen, if only because the nurses themselves enjoyed better health.

Although government district and central offices were moved from Herbertshöhe to Rabaul between October 1909 and January 1910, the hospital for Europeans was not ready. While awaiting its construction on the hillside at Namanula, the doctor treated Europeans at home and serious cases

144 Wendland, report 1.1.-31.3.1902, RKA 5729: 31

145 One room measured 4.9m x 4.6m, one 5.10m x 12m, and the third 5.10m x 3m. The fourth room, measuring 4.9m x 4.6m, was set up as a small laboratory and a dispensary. The fifth room, likewise 4.9m x 4.6m, was occupied by the nursing sister. Accommodation for the Chinese cook and the 'coloured' hospital attendants was in a separate outhouse, as were the kitchen, storeroom, laundry, bathroom and lavatory. The doctor's residence was close by. MB 1903/04: 178

146 MB 1907/08: 405-6

147 In 1904 Wendland mentions a particularly difficult patient, a big man, a heavy drinker, whose recovery was expected to take months following an operation for a complicated fracture of the femur. His nursing care would have been too much for the one nurse at the hospital. RKA 5729: 103

148 MB 1907/08: 406

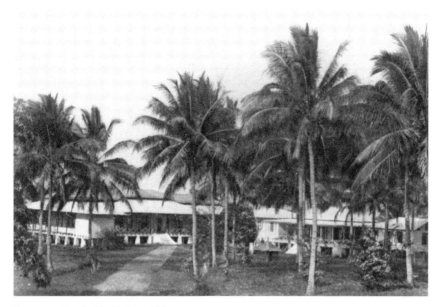

European Hospital in Herbertshöhe

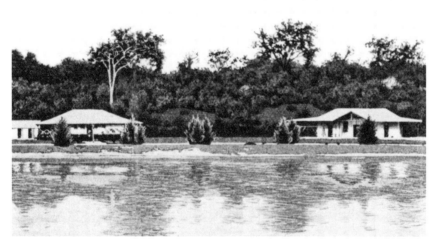

Residences of the government surveyor (left) and the government doctor (right),
Kaewieng, ca 1903

83

were transported to Herbertshöhe hospital.[149] The first stage of the new hospital complex in Rabaul was opened in April 1911. It consisted of a five-room main building offering accommodation for six patients, and an operating room and a laboratory. The nurses' residence was connected with the main hospital by a covered walkway. Kitchen, store rooms, sleeping quarters for hospital attendants, bathrooms, lavatories and laundries were in separate outhouses. The second stage, built during 1912, included an isolation ward and an operating theatre and a laboratory. This freed two of the rooms in the main building, which were turned into the 'women's wing' and increased the capacity to ten beds. With the opening of this hospital, the number of Red Cross nursing sisters for German New Guinea was increased from three to four, that is, two worked at the Rabaul hospital, one in Herbertshöhe, and one in Friedrich-Wilhelmshafen.[150]

That public pressure influenced the decision making process in deciding when to construct a hospital can be shown by the example of Kaewieng. A station was established there in 1900. It was not until the last quarter of 1903 that a doctor was sent there to organise medical facilities. One of his early requests was for a hospital for Europeans and a doctor's residence. At that time the number of settlers was small—four government employees, three of them married, plus managers of the various plantations, not usually married. A hospital could not be justified, although Hahl admitted that when it came to choosing the location for European housing and hospitals, "the best [was] barely good enough".[151] The doctor's residence was built, but the hospital had to wait. The need for a European hospital in Kaewieng was from then on highlighted repeatedly in medical reports, especially when there was a change in medical staff. By 1908 the number of European residents had increased to around forty—of whom eight were women and six children—hence the need was increasingly urgent.[152] In 1911 the Kaewieng District Office submitted another request. Hahl managed to resist the pressure, pointing to many more urgent needs: there were still stations without any medical staffing of any sort; setting up native hospitals had a high priority; a hospital was in any case a heavy long-term commitment by the government, one that was not justified in Kaewieng.[153] Patience among residents at Kaewieng —by then there were ninety-eight Europeans in the district, of which eighteen were women and twelve children—was running out at this stage and they formed a United

149 MB 1909/10: 476
150 MB 1910/11: 622; 1911/12: 480-81
151 Hahl to Danneil, G255/892: 1 ff

152 MB 1907/08: 445-6
153 Hahl to Boluminski, 14.10.1911, G255/892: 1b

Settlers Association to pressure the government to include a hospital in the next budget. Hahl was still not convinced.[154] The association decided to take direct action by starting up its own hospital fund and approaching the Patriotic Women's League[155] in Berlin for support. One of the reasons given for the need of a hospital was the lack of accommodation in Kaewieng for sick people from outlying areas, another the increasing number of women and children in Kaewieng and its surrounding areas, in particular the lack of a midwife.[156] The death of one woman in childbirth, a neonatal death, and a very long and difficult labour for the doctor's wife, resulting in a stillbirth,[157] demonstrated the need for a medical support system that also served women. The application was supported by district officer Boluminski, and signed by fifty-one settlers.[158] The direct application to the league had the desired effect and the Colonial Office agreed to add the sum of 30 000 Mark to the 1914 budget for a hospital in Kaewieng. As Hahl expected that this would be approved in the 1914 or the very latest the 1915 budget, he considered it inappropriate for the collection of private funds for the hospital to continue and suggested that the money collected so far be used to provide free hospital accommodation for needy settlers or for maternity cases.[159] War intervened before the proposed "Boluminski Hospital"[160] was built.

While it appears that the welfare of women and children living in the colony was a strong motivation for providing health care and hospital facilities, the absence of white women was an equal consideration. Unmarried plantation managers and government employees caused as much concern as

154 Hahl to Kirchner, 31.10.1912, G255/892: 1a
155 The Patriotic Women's League, under the patronage of the Empress, was the largest women's organisation in Wilhelmine Germany, with half a million members in 1910. Welfare work was one of its activities. Weindling 181
156 Hoffmann's letter of 22.9.1912, supporting the application to the Women's Association. G255/892: 2ff. In his memoirs Wendland recalled that the increased number of women and children required the setting up of a hospital in Rabaul. Wendland, *Im Wunderland der Papuas* (Berlin-Dahlem: Kurzeja) 164
157 MB 1909/10: 524; MB 1911/12: 524, 534
158 The first signature was that of Dr Hoffmann, followed by those of Mrs. Hoffmann, and the medical orderly Lachmann and his wife. Signatories also were the local managers of the plantation companies, a priest from the Catholic Mission, and other settlers in the Kaewieng district. The plan was for a small two-room hospital which would accommodate four patients, and an operating and treatment room, a house for a nursing sister, and the necessary ancillary buildings. Boluminski to Hahl, Application by Kaewieng Hospital Association to Women's Association in Berlin, 13.5.1913, G255/892: 2 ff
159 Hahl to District Officer Kaewieng 29.12.1913, G255/892: 15-16
160 Hahl supported the call by the Kaewieng residents that the new hospital be named in memory of the recently deceased District Officer Boluminski. G255/892: 15-16

married men and their families. An unmarried man was apt to take a native woman as housekeeper, and children were a likely result. Dr Runge found that such children had little resistance to disease, and half of them showed clear signs of "degeneracy". Strong tendencies to tuberculosis, symptoms of rickets, or congenital syphilis, were all indications that mixed-race children were of inferior quality and had a very short life expectancy. Concubinage with native women was therefore highly undesirable.[161] In his views on mixed-race children, Runge was clearly influenced by eugenic theories; a tendency to tuberculosis, rickets and congenital syphilis were among the 'racial diseases' much deplored by eugenicists.

The government could not directly intervene in the domestic affairs of an unmarried man, but it could create conditions which encouraged men to bring partners from Germany. Catering for the health needs of women and children was one such measure; adequate housing for families was another, both much advocated for doctors. Housing for government employees began to improve with the construction of Rabaul, but doctors remained concerned about a general housing shortage for families in the colony.[162]

Water Supply and Sanitation

Sanitation and water supply for settlers throughout the colony were such that with reasonable care dysentery and other intestinal diseases due to polluted water were not common in later years. For the capital, Governor Hahl's long term plans were to replace rainwater tanks with piped water and to build a sewage system and stormwater drains which would take waste water directly into the sea. The waste water system was to include all of Namanula and the Melanesian quarter.[163] Trials with earthenware pipes had shown that they withstood regular earth tremors. The Chinese quarter and the Botanical Garden were excluded on the grounds of costs. Piped water was to be brought to the houses in Namanula from a storage dam fed by a spring on the slopes of the "North Daughter". In downtown Rabaul piped water would mean the removal of the Norddeutscher Lloyd water storage tank, whose permanently damp surroundings were a well known mosquito breeding ground.

---

161 Runge, report 1.10.-31.12.1911, RKA 5772: 117; MB 1911/12: 503-4
162 Wick, RKA 5771: 132; MB 1911/12: 484-6
163 This would not only ensure a clean water supply and safe disposal of sanitary waste, but also help to reduce the number of mosquito breeding grounds around domestic rainwater tanks.

Not for the first time, plans were hampered by finances and Hahl had to find ways other than budgetary allocations from Berlin to fund the project. He started negotiations for the funding of these works by a public utilities company headed by Mertens, who was also the director of the Bismarck Archipelago Gesellschaft with plantations in New Ireland.[164] Negotiations were much slower than Hahl anticipated, and ran into difficulties when doubts were raised about the business integrity of Mertens,[165] so that by 1914 Rabaul was still without piped water or sewage and drainage systems.

Cost of Hospitals

Mention has been made of the high cost of running a European hospital. 'Housekeeping costs' for the Herbertshöhe hospital for 1905, when eighty-three patients were hospitalised, support this contention:[166]

Table 6
Hospital house-keeping costs

Item	Mark
food and drink	12,201
medications and bandaging materials	694
wages for 'coloured' hospital staff	1,092
food and other items for attendants and laundry and cleaning needs	1,320
Total	15,307

The salary for the nurse was paid in Germany by the Red Cross; the government paid 'pocket money' of 50 Mark per month, an amount not included in the hospital accounts. Apart from food and medications for patients, the hospital also provided meals for nurses; doctors and senior government employees could get board until they made their own domestic arrangements.[167] On this basis the expenditure for 1905 was 15,307 Mark, against an income from patients and boarders of 11,167 Mark. The hospital therefore had a deficit of 4,140 Mark on running costs alone. No allowance was made for depreciation and maintenance. Apart from the capital investment, the

---

164 Hahl to RKA 2.3.1908, RKA 5774: 3-7; Hahl to RKA 23.3.1909, RKA 2392: 37 ff
165 RKA 2393 and 2394
166 Accounts European Hospital Herbertshöhe, 1.4.1905-31.3.1906, G255/640
167 During the year two senior government officials and Dr Seibert had their board there for some months.

European hospital was a considerable annual cost to the government.

Government employees and their families were entitled to free medical treatment and hospitalisation, as were naval personnel in government hospitals. In this respect the hospital was part of the conditions of service for people in government employ. The Baining settlers were given free hospitalisation also. The remaining patients were charged a daily fee of 10 Mark in first class and 6 Mark in second class in 1904, a fee which was increased to 12 Mark and 7 Mark respectively in 1911.[168] In addition, there was a daily fee of 4 Mark for first class patients and 3 Mark for second class patients for medical consultations and treatment, payable to the doctor.[169] The daily hospital fee of 10 Mark represented roughly the cost of services provided, which in 1905 was about 9 Mark per patient per day.[170]

Food and drink, costing approximately 7 Mark per person per day, were by far the biggest expenditure, about four fifths of the running costs. Eggs, chicken, fresh fruit and vegetables and fresh fish were bought locally. Other supplies were all imported and they added up to a considerable list. The Norddeutscher Lloyd steamers brought in fresh meat, ham, and potatoes from Australia. Staples such as flour, sugar, coffee and tea, and many tinned foods such as fruit, fruit juices, vegetables, milk, butter, sauerkraut, geese breasts, and caviar were all imported. Wine, vermouth, port, madeira, beer, cider and soda water were also included in the hospital purchases. The pantry was well stocked to cater for the patients' jaded appetites. The bill for wages and food for labourers was around fifteen percent of the costs. The cost of medications and bandages was surprisingly small at less than five percent of the total. The care of the physical well-being of the patients with food and nursing seems to have been as important as medical treatment. Housekeeping at the hospital was certainly generous. The domestic staff, consisting of a Chinese cook, 'boys' for cleaning and gardening work and washerwomen, ensured smooth management.

Patients often stayed longer than strictly medical criteria warranted. It was a refuge for people from isolated settlements, so the wife of police sergeant

---

168 The increase occurred after costs had risen and accounting had become more realistic by including depreciation. *Amtsblatt* 1911: 173. Hospital costs and conditions for Europeans and natives were formalised in the *Bestimmungen des Gouverneurs von Deutsch-Neuguinea, betr. die Aufnahme und Behandlung in den Krankenhäusern des Gouvernements.* 25 July, 1911, *DKB* 22(1911): 201-2

169 RKA 5730: 76

170 This figure is arrived at by dividing the running cost for the year (less the fees paid by the boarders) by the number of days patients had spent in hospital (83 patients, total of 1492 days). G255/640

Fitsch, following a "perfectly normal delivery and no subsequent complications", stayed at the hospital for eight weeks.[171] For a while she could enjoy the company of other European women. People from the Baining Mountains were not always able to get transport home immediately, but no doubt appreciated the break from an isolated farm.

Medications and bandages cost 46 Pfennig per patient per day. The main pharmaceutical items used were antimalarial drugs, that is quinine in different forms, antiseptics, disinfectants, and analgesics and medications for ulcers and skin complaints. Bandages and absorbent cotton wool were other major items.

A comparison of running costs for European and native hospitals is revealing. In the years 1910 and 1911 the cost per patient per day in the Herbertshöhe native hospital was around 70 to 90 Pfennig; at Rabaul the cost was slightly higher at around 1 Mark. Included in this cost was food, medications and bandages, wages for medical orderlies and hospital attendants, a fraction of doctors' salaries, and maintenance and depreciation of buildings and equipment. Food costs were around 30 Pfennig per patient per day, medications and bandages around 35 Pfennig. Staple food for the hospitals, traded for tobacco from natives, but also purchased from small planters, was root crops and bananas, supplemented by rice, and tea and biscuits. Fresh pork and fish were served once or twice a week. Red and white wine was given to patients for medicinal purposes. Each patient was issued with a new loin cloth, tobacco and a pipe, and a blanket if none was brought along.[172]

The vast differences in costs was mainly due to the high costs of food served to Europeans. Food for native patients cost around 30 Pfennig, for a European patient it was more like 7 Mark, twenty-three times the cost. Costs of medications and bandaging material did not differ much with 46 Pfennig per day for a European, and 35 Pfennig for natives.[173] It seems there were no great differences in the pharmaceutical supplies used, with the exception of quinine. Europeans were given quinine in the expensive forms of capsules, tablets or injections; in the native hospital the far cheaper liquid quinine was the standard supply.[174]

A Hill Station

One way of restoring settlers to health was repatriation, another was a convalescence trip to the Gazelle-Peninsula, Singapore or Java. Both options were costly and depended on the availability of a ship. Therefore the New

171 Seibert, report 1.7.–31.10.1905, RKA 5769: 148
172 RKA 5731: 7 ff; G255/2
173 RKA 5731: 7ff
174 G255/639; 640. I am indebted to David Lowrey for elucidating the pharmaceutical supply lists.

Guinea Company sought ways of reducing costs, while at the same time providing a facility for colonists. A convalescent home at higher altitudes was
seen as of potentially great benefit to all and, with visions of an English-style
hill station, a search for a suitable location began. The disastrous year of 1891
seemed to make such a home urgent. But, despite repeated expressions of need
and concern, matters never went further. Considering the many problems
the company was facing, it should come as no surprise that nothing was done
during the 1890s. Ten years later the project was taken up seriously with a
proposal by the administrator of the New Guinea Company for the establishment of a health station in the hinterland of the Astrolabe Plain, ten kilometres inland from Stephansort, with funds to be requested from the Welfare
Lottery.[175] A contribution of 40,000 Mark from the lottery was approved.
The government was not happy with the location as it was in the middle of
the New Guinea Company plantations and would basically serve New
Guinea Company employees only. Hahl therefore suggested that the
Neuendettelsauer Mission build a convalescent home on Sattelberg with the
funds from the lottery. This would be more accessible, and its suitability was
proven through ten years' of occupancy.[176] Flierl declined on the grounds
that Sattelberg was not entirely malaria-free and that, because of very heavy
rain fall and thick fogs, it was suitable for convalescence only from
November to April.[177] Back in Berlin more research was done into the cost
of running such a station, only to rate it as too expensive for the relatively
few white people in the colony. A suggestion by the New Guinea Company
that the Rhenish Mission be given the funds to build a station on
Hansemannberg (north of Friedrich-Wilhelmshafen) was adopted instead; by
the end of 1903 clearing of grounds started and orders were placed in Sydney
for building materials.[178] Before much progress was made, Flierl announced

---

175 RKA 5802: 2-19, NGC to *Wohlfahrtslotterie* 16.12.1901. The *Wohlfahrtslotterie* was set up in
     1898 by the German Colonial Society and the German Women's Association for Nursing in
     the Colonies to raise money for developmental purposes in the colonies. Welfare Lottery tick-
     ets were sold throughout Germany. It was an indirect way of raising funds for colonial pur-
     poses which were not subject to Reichstag approval although no funds could be allocated
     without the consent of the Colonial Office. Money was allocated for a variety of purposes. In
     1899 funds were approved for the support of the scheme for the settling of German women
     in Southwest Africa; a contribution to the Tanganyika steamer scheme; contributions to sci-
     entific expeditions; the construction of a hospital in Tanga; examination of water resources in
     East Africa. *DKZ* 15 (1898): 417; 16(1899): 15
176 Hahl to Flierl 14.4.1903, RKA 5802: 79-80
177 Flierl to Hahl 27.4.1903, RKA 5802: 81 ff
178 RKA 5802: 87-11

that a modest three-roomed house to be used as a convalescent home had been completed on the Sattelberg to replace the primitive hut in which guests had previously been accommodated; any Europeans not needing medical attention were welcome to make use of it.[179] Immediately the government called for a reconsideration of the building at Hansemannberg which, in any case, could not be a substitute for a trip to Europe. The Hansemannberg project was therefore abandoned at the beginning of 1905[180] and with it the hope that a suitable site for a hill station would be found in Kaiser-Wilhelmsland in the foreseeable future.

In the Bismarck Archipelago, "the urgent necessity" for a convalescent home forced action a year later and Toma, some 40 kilometres from Rabaul, was chosen as the site. Hahl would have preferred to go higher up on the slopes of Vunakokor to about 500 metres, but did not consider such an isolated location safe enough. There would have been "considerable costs" in safeguarding such an advanced post. Toma was seen as a "reliable" district and had to be accepted as the best possible location for a sanatorium.[181] The residence of the police sergeant was converted and refurbished at a cost of 17,000 Mark, of which four fifths was paid by the Welfare Lottery. Eighteen months later Hahl disbanded the police station at Toma altogether, as he considered the natives in the surrounding areas to be completely pacified. The house built for the police sergeant in 1906 was refurbished, and additional outbuildings were constructed.[182] At long last the vision was fulfilled and the colony had its own hill station. All that remained was the setting up of house rules and conditions for admittance, and the purchase of two horses and an American buggy for the transport of guests. Both were readily forthcoming.[183] Funds for refurbishing and extending the hillstation were provided by the Welfare Lottery. The establishment proved very popular, so much so that at the beginning of 1914 the acting governor decided that the station needed further extensions as well as refurbishing and he again sought funds from the Welfare Lottery.[184] The Australians arrived too early to take advantage of any proposed improvements.

179 RKA 5802: 125
180 Meeting in Friedrich-Wilhelmshafen of Hahl, Stuckhardt, Dr Hoffmann, Loag and Sigwanz, RKA 5802: 145 ff
181 A police station had been established there in 1902 following the murder of Mrs. Wolff and her baby

182 RKA 5803: 40-41; 57 ff
183 House Rules for the home at Toma specified eligibility criteria, cost of transport, and for board and lodging. *Amtsblatt* 1910: 47
184 RKA 5803: 124

The need for good medical services for the newcomers became obvious from the beginning of settlement. Unless people enjoyed a standard of health which allowed them to work, the colony could not be developed. Yet the health factor was grossly misjudged and from this followed catastrophic miscalculations. The result was that many suffered severe ill health and other hardship, and many lost their lives prematurely, despite the presence of a doctor.

Medical services remained limited until the Reich took over the colony and the administration was moved to the Gazelle Peninsula. This meant that the European population centre was being established in a district with a much lower malaria endemicity than Friedrich-Wilhelmshafen, so that the move was a most important public health measure for the newcomers. Coincidentally the move to the Gazelle Peninsula happened at a time of advances in medical science by which malaria therapy and prophylaxis became possible with an appropriate quinine schedule. However, the hope that malaria could be eradicated was not fulfilled and, in order to further protect settlers, a policy of racial segregation was adopted. While malaria remained the main threat to the newcomers' health, venereal diseases also caused grave concern, as did tuberculosis, especially when its spread to the native population became obvious.

In keeping with the development of the capital, by 1914 considerable medical and hospital services had been set up there, and elsewhere planning was well advanced for improvements in the hospital services for the small number of newcomers. As befitted a hospital of a capital, the Rabaul hospital was well equipped and good care was provided; it was a model for other European hospitals to be built in the colony. It was also an object of pride, a symbol of the progress achieved since German rule began. New settlers could now expect to find health services similar to those at home—a most satisfactory situation. Whether the situation was as satisfactory for those who laboured for the European masters will be considered in the next chapter.

3

THE LABOUR FORCE

*...the exaggerated care for the welfare of labourers...
ruthlessly damages and neglects the interests of
planters.*[1]

This chapter examines two related questions concerning the labour force. The first one is an examination of labour mortality rates in German New Guinea and a comparison with other plantation colonies in the Pacific region at a similar stage of development.. The second is an examination of the trials and errors of the two colonial administrations in their endeavours to develop strategies and policies to bring about improvements in labourers' health. The focus is on the predominant and intractable problems: malaria and its prevention, dysentery and sanitation, and beriberi and nutrition.

MORTALITY RATES

Kaiser-Wilhelmsland

Labour mortality rates in German New Guinea have been the subject of a lively debate. In *New Guinea under the Germans*, Stewart Firth discussed morbidity and mortality among Asian coolies and Melanesian labourers in Kaiser-Wilhelmsland plantations in the 1890s to 1903. His verdict was that the price for plantation development had been "human suffering and death on a scale unknown on the British side of the island".[2] Sack, commenting on the monograph, argued that Firth had not provided enough detail on

---

1   Memorandum NGC to Colonial Office on proposed Labour Ordinance, 29.7.1914. RKA 2314: 8
2   Firth, *New Guinea* 43

mortality rates, and had over-emphasised the disasters of the early period and neglected the later period when mortality rates had dropped considerably.[3]

I have covered the same ground and used some additional material—but the question of the number of deaths during the first half of German colonisation of New Guinea remains unanswered. At best, what records are available allow an estimate of mortality rates over the years; as Firth pointed out, "Hahl himself was still searching for the answer in 1913".[4] It was highly unlikely that he was ever going to find a complete answer for, as Sister Hertzer noted at the end of 1891, "with six to eight labourers dying each day, they died uncounted".[5]

Importation of large numbers of coolies from the Dutch East Indies and the Straits Settlements to work on tobacco plantations began in the second half of 1891. Every single one became infected with malaria and, in combination with dysentery, it was fatal for many in the first few months. Of 313 Chinese who arrived at the end of September 1891 over a quarter had died within three months.[6] About 1840 coolies arrived in Kaiser-Wilhelmsland between September 1891 and March 1892.[7] By 30 June 1892 there were only 950 left, suggesting that 890 (48 per cent) had died within a short time of arrival. The mortality may be even higher as only 220 coolies were in Kaiser-Wilhelmsland on 1 January 1891.[8] We do not know whether they were part of the 950 still there on 30 June 1892. If so, it would mean that around 1100 coolies (53 per cent) died in 18 months from January 1891 to June 1892. Firth's calculations of 988 Chinese having arrived within eight months from August 1891 to March 1892, with only 420 left in Kaiser-Wilhelmsland indicates a similar percentage of Chinese dying (57 per cent).[9] Imperial Commissioner Rose estimated that by mid-1892 well over one third of the coolies had died, and that most of the others were dying.[10]

It is not possible to establish rates of death for Melanesians. Little data is available for the first few years, or for 1891, the confused times when "all people [were] going around as if they were not quite right in their head, Europeans and natives alike".[11] Rose estimated that at least 15 per cent of all

3 P. Sack, 'A History of German New Guinea: A Debate about Evidence and Judgement,' *JPH* 20.2(1985): 84-94

4 S. Firth, 'German New Guinea: The Archival Perspective,' *JPH* 20.2(1985): 94-103: 101

5 Hertzer diary 20 December 1891

6 Rose report to Chancellor von Caprivi, 24.12.1891, RKA 2980: 196

7 *NKWL* 1892: 31 (1085 Chinese and 757 Javanese). Firth, *New Guinea* 35 quotes a figure of around 1700; RKA 2427: 143ff, 160, Astrolabe Company reports)

8 Rose report 30.6.1892, RKA 6512: 45 ff

9 Firth, *New Guinea* 35

10 Rose report 30.6.1892, RKA 6512: 52

11 Hertzer diary 19 December 1891

Table 7
Labour mortality rate, Friedrich-Wilhelmshafen 1892-1896

Year	Av. no of labourers	No of deaths	Annual rate per thousand
1892 (9 months)	226	37	218
1893	270	68	251
1894	265	46	173
1895	293	29	98
1896	222	26	117

Melanesian labourers had died in the influenza epidemic in November and December 1891.[12] The number probably rose, as the epidemic did not abate until February 1892.[13] Mortality in Friedrich-Wilhelmshafen, where the labour force was almost entirely Melanesian, is set out in Table 7 above.[14]

Snippets of information suggest an annual mortality rate of up to 25 per cent for Stephansort for the years 1892-95.[15] The number of deaths among Melanesians during a smallpox epidemic in the second half of 1893 in Stephansort was never published by the company. Judge Krieger, who arrived in Stephansort towards the end of 1893, noted that 351 Melanesian labourers had died in Stephansort from smallpox.[16] Influenza followed smallpox, decimating the Melanesian labour force again between October and December 1894. At the same time beriberi began to make an impact. In the twelve months to November 1894, 245 men came down with beriberi,[17] and in the year to March 1896 of the 137 beriberi patients eighty-seven, nearly two out of three, died. The number of Melanesians with beriberi as a percentage of the total number of Melanesian labourers increased: while 2 per cent had been affected in 1893/94, in the following year 7.4 per cent suffered from beriberi.[18] With an average 1,695 labourers[19] in Stephansort, the eighty-seven deaths represent a beriberi mortality rate of 51.3 per thousand. For the year

12 Rose report 24.12.1891, RKA 2980: 195 ff
13 Internal memorandum of AA, RKA 2981: 16
14 Calculated from Dempwolff report, RKA 5769: 11 -12 and 'Aerztliche Erfahrungen' 281
15 Hagen noted that following repatriation of chronic and incurable cases, morbidity fell in 1896/7 to between 7 and 8 per cent, a third of previous years. Hagen 35
16 M. Krieger, 1899, *Neu-Guinea* (Berlin: Schall, 1899) 177-8
17 Hagen, op. cit 39, 43
18 W. Wendland, 'Ueber das Auftreten der Beri-Beri Krankheit in Kaiser-Wilhelmsland,' *ASTH* 1 (1897): 241
19 From April to December 1895 there were on average 518 Chinese, 553 Javanese and 624 Melanesians in Stephansort. AR 1894/95: 113

to February 1896 the company acknowledged that, out of an average force of 1956 labourers, 540 had died, a death rate of 276 per thousand.[20]

Although repatriation of all 'unfit' coolies brought about a reduction in deaths after April 1896, diarrhoeal diseases persisted: throughout the year there were sporadic cases of dysentery and an epidemic of gastroenteritis claimed twenty-seven lives, about one fifth of the 125 deaths. For the year 1896/97 mortality was about 76 per thousand,[21] a rate further reduced in the following year to around 30 per thousand.[22] 1897/98 was perhaps atypical as the number of labourers dropped to around 750 early in 1898, the lowest number for several years. Only those who had withstood the prevalent diseases were still there. Furthermore, during that period only ninety Melanesians were recruited but no coolies.[23]

The situation in Stephansort changed rapidly when a shipment of 266 Chinese coolies arrived from Macao in the last days of December 1898. Within one month about half of them were hospitalised; four died in January and another thirty-eight in February, malaria and dysentery being the main causes. There were many deaths among Melanesians, affected also by malaria and dysentery. In the year to September 1899 there were 201 deaths at Stephansort. With an average of 790 labourers on the station, the mortality rate was 254 per thousand. Well over a hundred of these deaths were Chinese coolies; around fifty were Melanesians. For the same period the situation in Friedrich-Wilhelmshafen was much better with a death rate of 43 per thousand.[24] The total labour force in Kaiser-Wilhelmsland during 1898/99 averaged 928; with a total of 207 deaths, the mortality rate was 223 per thousand. This was the last year with extremely high rates of over two hundred deaths per thousand labour population.

A considerable drop in the death rate to 75 per thousand occurred in 1899/1900, when Professor Koch spent some months in Kaiser-Wilhelmsland experimenting with malaria eradication. A systematic quininisation program can be credited with contributing to a decrease in deaths.

In April 1901 about two hundred coolies were brought in from Swatow in southern China, and most were stationed in Friedrich-Wilhelmshafen.

---

20 NGC to AA 29.5.1896, RKA 2985: 109
21 AR 1896/97: 133; *NKWL* 1898: 27
22 *NKWL* 1897: 26 ff
23 Recruitment had come to a near standstill as no shipping was available following the sinking of the *Johann Albrecht. NKWL* 1898:24
24 AR 1898/9: 162-3, 166

Mortality rose again with forty-eight Chinese dying within the next six months. For the year to September 1901 there were on average 605 labourers in Friedrich-Wilhelmshafen of whom seventy-two died, a mortality rate of 119 per thousand. In the period October 1900 to March 1901 there were, on average, eighty-six Chinese on Friedrich-Wilhelmshafen station, of whom three died, a mortality rate of 35 per thousand for the six months' period. In the following six months, with the April intake, there were on average 278 Chinese on the station, of whom forty-eight died, a death rate of 173 per thousand. These figures typify the variation within a twelve months period with a death rate in one half roughly five times higher than in the other. Of the seventy-two deaths 44 per cent were due to beriberi among new arrivals, and 28 per cent to dysentery.

Unlike earlier years, health conditions in the year to March 1901 were better in Stephansort than in Friedrich-Wilhelmshafen. Out of an average of 410 labourers on the station, thirty-nine died, a mortality rate of 95 per thousand. Of the thirty-nine dead two thirds were Melanesians, a death rate of 98 per thousand for an average of 265 Melanesians. Of the average of seventy-nine Chinese, thirteen died, a death rate of 165 per thousand. None of the sixty-six Javanese on the station died. Seventeen of the thirty-nine deaths were due to dysentery, and only one to beriberi.[25]

During 1901 the labour force in Kaiser-Wilhelmsland was greatly reduced. On average only three hundred labourers were in Stephansort of whom twenty-four died, a mortality rate of 80 per thousand. In Friedrich-Wilhelmshafen forty-one died from an average of 566, a mortality rate of 72 per thousand.[26]

Paradoxically, despite better documentation and reporting after the Reich took over the administration of the colony, it is difficult to establish mortality rates for the second period of German colonisation of Kaiser-Wilhelmsland. Reports from the government doctor in the company hospital in Friedrich-Wilhelmshafen were not compiled regularly.[27] There is also no way of establishing the size of the "population at risk". We know the number of deaths at that hospital, but have little information to relate them to a population group. There were labourers employed by the company in the Friedrich-Wilhelmshafen district, with the main contingent from its Yomba plantations. From other stations, such as Stephansort, with a sizeable labour force, seriously ill patients were transferred to the Friedrich-Wilhelmshafen hospital. The hospi-

25 AR NGC 1900/01: 23-24, RKA 2419: 18-19, 22 ff
26 AR NGC 1901/02: 16, RKA 2419: 22 ff
27 No reports submitted when doctor was on leave and a locum replaced him.

tal catered also for people in government employ—police troops and labourers—
and convicts sentenced to forced labour in Friedrich-Wilhelmshafen.

The following example demonstrates the difficulty. During 1903/04 there
were twenty-eight deaths in Friedrich-Wilhelmshafen hospital: seventeen
were labourers from the local New Guinea Company plantation. The annual average number of labourers was 421, therefore the mortality rate was 40
per thousand for this group of labourers. The remainder came from the following places: five men returned from an expedition in the Huon Gulf; three
from Stephansort plantations; two from other company stations, and one
from a ship's crew.[28] There is no information on Stephansort or other stations, nor on the size of the Huon Gulf expeditionary force. It is clearly
impossible to calculate mortality rates other than for the Friedrich-
Wilhelmshafen plantation. The situation becomes more complicated still in
the following years with deaths of convicts. Of the eight deaths among 'government people' in 1904/05, six were convicts; most of the ten deaths in the
next year were convicts, and so were the nine in 1909/10.[29] These figures
suggest that for many convicts the sentence to hard labour in Kaiser-
Wilhelmsland was a death sentence.

Bismarck Archipelago

In the Bismarck Archipelago, mortality rates of New Guinea Company
plantation labourers were considerably lower than in Kaiser-Wilhelmsland,
as figures from 1896 to 1903 show (Table 8, page 99).[30]

For the remainder of the German period a calculation of the mortality rate
in the Bismarck Archipelago is beset by the same difficulties as for Kaiser-
Wilhelmsland. Furthermore, police troops from the Caroline Islands were
often accompanied by families, so that the population pool is even wider and
more disparate than in Kaiser-Wilhelmsland. Deaths of such family members
were included in labour statistics.

Table 9 (page 99, below) shows that labour mortality rates differed considerably between plantations of the main firms based on the Gazelle Peninsula.[31]

28 MB 1903/4: 255
29 The six convicts who died in 1904/5 were from the Baining Mountains, sentenced to hard
    labour after the Baining Massacre. (MB 1904/5: 166). More Baining prisoners died in the
    following year. (MB 1905/6: 279) No identification of the 1909/10 prison deaths. (MB
    1909/10: 479)
30 Calculated from figures in the AR NGC.
31 Hahl to RKA 9.3.1913, RKA 2313: 89. For the purpose of this exercise, missions are treated
    as plantation firms.

Table 8
Labour mortality rate, Bismarck Archipelago 1896–1903

Year	Av. no. labourers	No. of deaths	Deaths per thousand
1896/97	601	30	49.9
1897/98	673	24	35.6
1898/99	579	10	17.3
1899/1900	852	55	64.5
1900/01	981	38	38.7
1901/02	1100	69	62.7
1902/03	1046	38	36.3

If these two years are typical for the whole period, it suggests that Mouton & Company had the worst record, with death rates for 1910 nearly three times as high as the average and nearly twice as high in 1911. It also goes some way towards supporting the frequent contention by doctors that some employers waited too long before they had sick labourers hospitalised. Quite often men were at the point of death by the time they were transferred to a government hospital. This practice ensured that labourers did not die on the plantation, something to be avoided as it brought a plantation into disrepute. The mortality rate of the largest employer, the New Guinea Company, with about 40 per cent of the labour force, was just below the average in 1910, and virtually identical with the average in 1911. The second largest employer, Forsayth & Company, was above average in both years. The Catholic Mission fared slightly better and the record of the Wesleyan Mission is quite remarkable.

Labour force mortality rates in Kaiser-Wilhelmsland and the Bismarck

Table 9
Labour mortality rate Gazelle Peninsula plantations 1910 and 1911

	1910			1911		
	Labourers	No of deaths	Per thousand	Labourers	No of deaths	Per thousand
NGC	1977	35	17.7	1902	52	27.3
Forsayth Co.	1235	34	27.5	1225	35	28.6
Rondahl	246	7	28.5	399	12	30.0
Mouton & Co.	195	11	56.4	210	11	52.4
Cath.Mission	778	6	7.7	832	19	22.8
Wesl.Mission	152	1	6.6	178	1	5.6
Total/Average	4583	94	20.5	4746	130	27.4

Archipelago combined for the years 1903-1913 ranged between 13 and 63 per thousand.[32] These figures suggest that the death rate had stabilised at a more acceptable level although there was undoubtedly room for improvement.

Reviewing the figures and statistics quoted so far, a mortality pattern similar to that of other plantation colonies emerges: high rates of death in the early years were followed by a gradual decline. However, as Table 10 shows, in German New Guinea mortality rates in the first years were much higher than at a similar stage of plantation development in Queensland and Fiji. They declined to a comparable level after roughly fifteen years, roughly corresponding to the time it took for a decline in labour mortality in Queensland and Fiji. It is notable, that the average mortality rate is virtually identical for Papua and New Guinea from 1902-1913, with 34.6 per thousand for Papua and 34 per thousand for German New Guinea.[33]

The decline in mortality rates in New Guinea is pronounced; starting with much higher figures than Queensland and Fiji, the reduction to levels comparable to other plantation economies is striking.

Shlomowitz's calculation of mortality rates for German New Guinea, based on the total number of recruits from the Bismarck Archipelago between 1887 and 1903, who died in Kaiser-Wilhelmsland or the Bismarck Archipelago during their indenture, is especially useful as a comparison. The death rate of 172 per thousand for Kaiser-Wilhelmsland, and 45 for the Bismarck Archipelago,[34] confirms the very high rates suggested in the above tables.

Whether the death rate in Kaiser-Wilhelmsland of local recruits was as high as it was of those recruited in the Bismarck Archipelago as Firth suggests,[35] is debatable. On the whole local recruits were far less prone to malaria as they were more or less immune to it. They were, of course, affected by dysentery and the disastrous smallpox and influenza epidemics. Yabim from the Finschhafen district were considered to be the healthiest labourers, inured to the vagaries of the climate, and therefore excellent recruits.[36] Experience confirmed in 1896/07 that recruits from Kaiser-Wilhelmsland were far more resistant to disease, with a morbidity and mortality rate only half that of those

32 Statistic compiled by Dr Wick, RKA 5773: 52 attachment
33 Sources: for Fiji: Shlomowitz, 'Mortality and the Pacific Labour Trade,' JPH 22.1/2 (1987): 48. For Papua: Shlomowitz, 'Mortality and Indentured labour in Papua (1885-1914) and New Guinea (1920-1941),' JPH 23.1 (1988): 70-7: 72; for Queensland: Shlomowitz, 'Pacific Labour Trade' 50. For German New Guinea: NKWL, AR, RKA
34 Shlomowitz, 'Pacific Labour Trade' 54
35 Firth, New Guinea 175
36 Hagen 38; Annual Report Astrolabe Co. 1893-94: 6, RKA 2428

Table 10
Comparison of labour mortality rates in plantation colonies

Queensland		Fiji		Papua		German New Guinea	
Year	Rate	Year	Rate	Year	Rate	Year	Rate
1870	n.a.	1879	51.1	-	-	1886	n.a.
1871	n.a.	1880	92.3	-	-	1887	n.a.
1872	n.a.	1881	45.6	-	-	1888	n.a.
1873	n.a.	1882	108.1	-	-	1889	n.a.
1874	n.a	1883	78.8	-	-	1890	n.a.
1875	85.1	1884	120.0	-	-	1891	n.a.
1876	63.7	1885	86.9	-	-	1892	21
1877	51.4	1886	49.8	-	-	1893	251
1878	n.a.	1887	n.a.	-	-	1894	173
1879	n.a.	1888	49.5	-	-	1895	276
1880	62.9	1889	56.4	-	-	1896	67
1881	64.7	1890	86.6	-	-	1897	32
1882	82.6	1891	44.9	-	-	1898	144
1883	75.3	1892	108.3	-	-	1899	70
1884	147.7	1893	104.2	-	-	1900	74
1885	98.8	1894	87.3	-	-	1901	68
1886	61.4	1895	63.0	1902/3	26	1902	38
1887	60.6	1896	22.9	1903/4	73	1903	41
1888	62.1	1897	9.3	1904/5	14	1904	31
1889	55.6	1898	7.4	1905/6	35	1905	27
1890	48.1	1899	14.6	1906/7	22	1906	25
1891	57.3	1900	25.4	1907/8	22	1907	13
1892	41.0	1901	5.5	1908/9	32	1908	32
1893	52.6	1902	8.4	1909/10	74	1909	34
1894	42.5	1903	47.6	1910/11	46	1910	35
1895	35.2	1904	25.8	1911/12	35	1911	29
1896	35.6	1905	22.9	1912/13	24	1912	63
1897	32.2	1906	15.9	1913/14	13	1913	40

from the Bismarck Archipelago.[37] Early in the century local recruits were reported as enjoying a much better state of health than those from the Bismarck Archipelago, as they suffered little from malaria,[38] and were therefore much sought after.

HEALTH POLICIES AND STRATEGIES

When the New Guinea Company undertook the colonisation of New Guinea and began its settlement in Finschhafen, public health issues were not much of a consideration. Alcohol was seen as the greatest health threat to the indigenous population and its sale to natives was therefore banned, together with a ban on the sale of weapons and ammunition.[39] This ban, similar to one applied by the British government in 1879 to Tonga, Samoa, Rotuma, and Niue, and in 1884 to Fiji,[40] constituted the company's public health policy at the beginning of colonisation. The next policy document came five years later when the high incidence of venereal infection in labourers recruited in the Bismarck Archipelago, especially among women, had repercussions among company men and labourers alike. In order to contain venereal disease, not only on stations but also in villages when labourers returned, medical examination of all Melanesian labourers was made compulsory.[41] It was the beginning of a battle that was still being waged in 1914.

Meantime, the company's decision to develop plantations in Kaiser-Wilhelmsland had serious implications for the health and welfare of the labour force. Labourers were imported without thought for their impact on the health of the native population or vice versa. The company wanted a labour force; instead it got people who created all manner of problems with their

37 NKWL 1897: 27
38 Hoffmann, MB 1903/4: 233
39 Erlass des Reichskanzlers betr. Landerwerbung in Kaiser-Wilhelmsland, Verbot der Abgabe von Waffen und Munition und Spirituosen an Eingeborene, Arbeiterausführung von Kaiser-Wilhelmsland und Bismarck Archipel. 8 June 1885. NKWL 1885(1): 5

40 D. Scarr, Fragments of Empire (Canberra: ANU Press, 1967) 162 (note) and 189
41 Verordnung betr. die gesundheitliche Kontrolle der im Schutzgebiet der Neu Guinea Kompagnie als Arbeiter angeworbenen Eingeborenen, 18. Oktober 1890. RKA 2301: 81-2. See also Firth, New Guinea 30, on the difficulties Imperial Commissioner Rose had with this ordinance.

high morbidity and mortality. Doctors were employed to keep the labourers healthy but failed in the first half of the German period. Rates dropped considerably after the turn of the century, and it bears examination whether this was due to medical intervention. While doctors were reluctant to accept responsibility for morbidity and mortality, they nevertheless had to find explanations. In the main these centred on the climate and its influence on health, the capacities of labourers to adapt to new conditions, and the failure of administrations or planters to follow doctors' advice.

The first doctor was highly optimistic: "There is no reason to have any serious reservations about colonising the country from the point of view of health. Rather it is to be hoped that with the increasing consolidation of conditions, more will be done in regard to hygiene and medical services and satisfactory progress would not fail to eventuate."[42] Alas, Schellong had to revise his views when health in Finschhafen did not improve and was equally poor on other stations. The explanation he offered was repeated by his successors many times: the relationship between the climate and the general state of health, in particular the incidence of malaria, and the capacity of newcomers to adapt to the climate.

Comparisons of climatic conditions revealed no hard and fast rules, except that climatic influences affected people at all times. In Finschhafen there were fewer malaria attacks during the dry months of March and April.[43] Seasonal changes increased the incidence of malaria. Occupation also had a bearing on well-being, with earth work (digging ditches, clearing work) proving particularly harmful to health.[44] In Stephansort malaria incidence was found to be highest during the dry season, such as the six months to October 1896, when there were 195 cases of malaria hospitalised of whom nineteen died; in the wet period, October 1896 to March 1897, there were 106 malaria patients with four deaths.[45] There was one point of general agreement: the likelihood that the "malign effects of the peculiarities of the climate" would affect all people for several more years[46] and that all new recruits had to undergo their "acclimatisation malaria".[47] Despite conflicting evidence, weather recording continued with great assiduity in the hope that eventually a clear relationship could be established between climatic conditions and the occurrence of one disease or another.

With the theory of racial differences in physiological functioning under

42 Schellong's report for the first half year. *NKWL* 1886: 128 ff
43 *NKWL* 1886: 131
44 *NKWL* 1890: 29, 31–35
45 *NKWL* 1897: 28
46 AR 1891–93: 82
47 Hagen 28

given climatic conditions foremost in mind and the hope that a race of people could be found that would readily adapt, the incidence of diseases among
the various racial groups was constantly monitored. The results were invari-
ably the same: Asian coolies were more prone to malaria than Melanesians.
The latter were certainly not immune as had been assumed, but the degree of
susceptibility varied. Young people from the Bismarck Archipelago and
Solomon Islanders were particularly prone to malaria, while local recruits and
'old hands' from New Britain suffered only occasional attacks.[48]

One of the first detailed morbidity reports published proved to be typical of many more to come: in the second half of 1890 in Finschhafen, forty-
three Javanese were hospitalised totalling eighty-eight cases, and 261
Melanesians totalling 297 cases,[49] which meant that on average each
Javanese was hospitalised twice, and that there were some multiple hospi-
talisations among Melanesians also. Nine out of ten Javanese cases were in
hospital because of malaria, compared with four out of ten Melanesians.
Only serious malaria cases were hospitalised, so the incidence of malaria was
much higher than these figures suggest. However, the figures also show the
high incidence of malaria among Melanesians who continued to surprise
doctors with their lack of immunity. Nearly a quarter of Melanesians were
hospitalised for "surgical"[50] conditions, forty-seven for the treatment of skin
problems, thirty-two for venereal and twenty for diarrhoeal diseases, six
for bronchial catarrh, and two for eye infections. For the first time in
medical reports beriberi and pulmonary tuberculosis were mentioned: one
Javanese was hospitalised with beriberi and one Melanesian with tuberculosis. As the years went by, causes of hospitalisation remained much the same,
although the number of patients treated for particular conditions varied a
great deal.

The weather was seen to have many other effects on health, be it respiratory tract infections, leg ulcers or dysentery. A dysentery epidemic in
Stephansort at the end of September 1889 was attributed to wet weather, and
similarly in Hatzfeldhafen, where the epidemic broke out in November 1889
and was brought under control only with the onset of the dry season in April,
after it had claimed nineteen lives.[51]

The first outbreak of dysentery was reported from Constantinhafen in mid-
1888. It was claimed that it was introduced from the neighbouring villages of

48 *NKWL* 1890: 27-38
49 *NKWL* 1891: 22
50 "surgical" was a broad group of condi-

tions, such as ulcers, abscesses, buboes, tissue inflammations and similar complaints.
51 *NKWL* 1890: 37-38; 87-88

Bongu, Kurenar and Gumbu where it had taken many victims.[52] There is no way of finding out whether the source of infection was in one of the villages or how it got there in the first place; or if in fact it was introduced from the villages to the stations, rather than the other way around. What is important is that it signalled the introduction of an infectious disease which spread rapidly.[53] It was never eradicated during the German period, and was a clear indication of poor sanitary conditions on stations. The first outbreak affected the whole station population, as was the case in the next few years, quite unlike epidemics in later years when colonists were affected to a much lesser degree. Dysentery outbreaks in these early years when the number of people on a station was relatively small, were a warning sign of problems to come. As events proved, the warning was ignored.

While there was little publicity about deaths among labourers in Kaiser-Wilhelmsland during the first few years of company rule, questions were asked in Germany about the high mortality following large scale importation of coolies. While "climatic influences" were still crucial, this explanation alone did not have sufficient force and the focus of attention had to be shifted. An "independent expert", a doctor on the Norddeutscher Lloyd steamer *Lübeck*, expressed the opinion that malaria was no more virulent in Friedrich-Wilhelmshafen than in other tropical countries. It was not malaria that was the problem, but the coolies, who had little resistance because of their "weaker constitution, traditional nutrition, and opium consumption".[54] Poor selection standards in Singapore[55] resulted in "wholesale importation of labourers of extremely inferior quality". When Hagen arrived in Stephansort he confirmed his colleague's opinion; the labour force was a "decrepit anaemic rabble" most of whom had never done plantation work before, "opium-weakened scum gathered in the streets of Singapore, inveterate opium smokers with little resistance to disease and therefore killed off quickly". Of eighty-five Chinese who arrived in Kaiser-Wilhelmsland on the same ship as Hagen, thirty-two died within three months. According to the doctor's diagnosis, only seven of these deaths were directly attributable to malaria, but twenty to opium smoking. His judgment that twenty-nine men were at the point of death on arrival in the colony had been quickly confirmed.[56]

---

52 *NKWL* 1888:182
53 An outbreak occurred around the same time on Hatzfeldhafen station, followed by outbreaks in Stephansort, with labourers succumbing on each station. *NKWL* 1889: 26; 1890: 37
54 Annual Report Astrolabe Co 1892/93: 7, RKA 2427; AR 1891-93: 81
55 AR 1891-92 and 1892-93: 81
56 Hagen 35-7

Hagen arrived in Stephansort three years after the Astrolabe Company had begun importing large numbers of coolies. Accommodation and hospital facilities had been improved, yet morbidity and mortality among new arrivals remained high. There was great need to find explanations that shifted attention from the company and from malaria.

The first five coolie transports were accompanied by ex-Sumatra planters[57]—they knew what type of people were required and were unlikely to accept people considered unsuitable. Opium consumption was probably taken for granted by Sumatra planters. While the company was able to depict the opium habit as affecting adaptation to Kaiser-Wilhelmsland, at the same time measures were taken quietly by introducing legislation so that coolies were able to purchase opium legally, which in turn ensured that they would continue to work and that others could be recruited.[58] The first contingents of coolies arriving in Kaiser-Wilhelmsland were therefore unlikely to be "scum" as they were described in 1893 and 1894, when recruitment had become very difficult and undoubtedly many coolies brought in were in very poor health. "Opium-enervated" had a lot of emotive force, and conflating this term with the description of later recruits—a conflation made easier by belated reporting[59]—created an impression that all coolies recruited for Kaiser-Wilhelmsland were in poor health on arrival.

This convenient explanation glossed over the conditions that awaited the first shipments of coolies. There was no proper accommodation, let alone sanitary facilities or provisions for the care of the sick.[60] Medications had to be used sparingly as stock was insufficient.[61] Despite the fact that doctors had established that all Asian labourers suffered severely from malaria and many would need hospitalisation, preparations for newcomers were, to say the least, inadequate.

The high incidence of beriberi was also explained by reference to the coolies' condition. Many had suffered from beriberi before coming to Kaiser-

---

57   Pfaff with the first transport in *Schwalbe* in September 1891, Puttkammer with *Nierstein* in the second in October 1891, Hanneken in third in December 1891 with *Devawongse*, fourth transport in *Nierstein* in January 1892, fifth transport with *Devawongse* with Rohlack in March 1892. Von Puttkammer was probably not a tobacco planter, but he had been there on a study tour and had some idea what tobacco coolies looked like.

58   Rose to AA 23.12.1890, RKA 2535: 4 ff; Verordnung betr. die Beschränkung und Beaufsichtigung der Einfuhr und des Vertriebs des Opiums im Schutzgebiet der Neu Guinea Kompanie, 30 December 1891. RKA 2964:134-5

59   See Sack and Clark, 1979, 'Introduction' to *German New Guinea: The Annual Reports*: xi

60   W. von Hanneken, 1895, 'Eine Kolonie in der Wirklichkeit', *Die Nation* 13(9):133-36; (10): 154-157, RKA 2983

61   Rose to AA 24.12.1891, RKA 2980: 198

Wilhelmsland; the indelible blue stamp on their lower back, applied to beriberi-patients by the army in the Dutch East Indies so that they could not be recruited again for military service, was ample proof. As they were not employable in Singapore and the Dutch East Indies because of this stamp, they engaged for work in Kaiser-Wilhelmsland where a relapse sooner or later was unavoidable.[62] Comparisons with coolie deaths on tobacco plantations in Sumatra, where mortality had been very high also, were further proof in the case against coolies.[63]

Once the explanation of the physical inadequacy of one racial group was accepted, it could be extended to others, as Hagen unwittingly demonstrated. The 306 men from New Hanover and New Ireland who arrived in mid-1894 all came down with malaria, and many were so sick that by October 144 of the group were hospitalised. When influenza broke out in October, about two thirds of the group succumbed. They were described as "exceptionally inferior people"— about one third had been unfit for work on arrival but the company had refused to repatriate them.[64]

Doctors connected physical condition and resistance to disease with race, whether for "opium-enervated" coolies or for "inferior" Melanesians. This preoccupation with race blinded doctors and the company to the fundamental problems of moving people from one epidemiological environment to another where they were exposed to new diseases, and unsanitary conditions were created by amassing people without adequate sanitation. While tolerable in a traditional life style, the lack of sanitation and clean water were catastrophic when large numbers of people were crowded together.

Because these basic questions were not addressed, each group of new arrivals encountered severe health problems, despite improved housing and the construction of hospitals. In Stephansort and in Friedrich-Wilhelmshafen native hospitals were built in 1892, but only after hundreds of labourers had died in the most appalling conditions in 1891. This raises the question whether there were not enough healthy people there to start construction any earlier, so that the company had to wait for people to get well before they could build a hospital.

The Friedrich-Wilhelmshafen complex consisted of wooden atap covered barracks, a large one as the men's ward, a smaller one as the women's ward, a mortuary, kitchen and laundry. Inside the men's ward was a freestanding platform built on 1.5 meter high pillars, accessible by three sets of stairs. On

---

62 Hagen 43

63 *NKWL* 1894: 27; Hagen 42-45

64 Hagen 29-30; 39

it stood rows of 1 meter high plank-beds which served also as transportable stretchers. Each bed had a mat, a blanket and a mosquito net. Along one wall of the barrack a number of rooms served as doctor's office, dispensary and storage. The barrack was seen as very suitable for its purpose: it was cool and light, each bed was readily accessible from all sides, and cleaning and disinfection was easy. The women's hospital was smaller with portable plank-beds placed on the paved floor. Sanitary facilities were minimal, and all sanitary waste was tipped straight into the sea, as was the case on the whole station, where "the tides took care of cleanliness". An isolation ward for dysentery and beriberi patients was set up on an uninhabited island. This was a simple shelter consisting of a few upright posts supporting an atap roof. Cooking facilities were under a similar shelter on bare ground. The grandly titled "quarantine station" on Piawey Island was identical.[65]

Hospitals were of course important, but they did not solve fundamental health problems or contribute to the prevention of disease. This was again demonstrated when around two hundred "carefully chosen, fit" Chinese arrived from Swatow for work in Friedrich-Wilhelmshafen in April 1901. Despite their "exceptionally good physical condition" and a reduction in the incidence of malaria, they fell ill and fifty-one died during the year, about half of them of beriberi and many of dysentery. The high mortality convinced the company that Chinese, "often afflicted with hereditary diseases", were unable to withstand the climate of the New Guinea littoral.[66]

With about seven out of ten deaths due to beriberi and dysentery, the evidence suggests that sanitation and nutrition were still neglected. The malaria prophylaxis program initiated by Professor Koch could not be carried out to the doctor's satisfaction either. Following Koch's instruction, Dr Hintze prescribed one gram of liquid quinine every ninth and tenth day, a dosage which kept the number of cases down and also reduced the virulence of attacks. The difficulty lay in ensuring that all labourers were given quinine regularly. Their numbers fluctuated considerably and labourers were shifted from one plantation to another. Station managers failed to keep the doctor informed of changes, and his instructions were forgotten; unless he went to the plantations personally on 'quinine days', the dosage was not handed out.[67] Yet, despite laxity, unsanitary conditions and poor nutrition, the company succeeded in placing blame neatly on the victims.

65   Dempwolff, 'Aerztliche Erfahrungen,' 138-9
66   AR NGC 1900/01: 18, RKA 2419: 22 ff
67   Private letter of Hintze to Koch 22.1.1902. Archives Robert-Koch-Institut

That the 'inferior quality' of recruits was a cause of high labour morbidity and mortality was asserted also in later years. A considerable number of recruits were reported as physically unfit for plantation labour; "weaklings, men chronically ill or infected with venereal disease, even cripples" signed on, either because villagers forced them so as to get rid of "a useless mouth" or in the hope that they would be cured when joining the labour force. Following a medical examination of all newly indentured recruits, about 10 per cent of them had to be hospitalised, but most of that group were considered to be fit for work after medical treatment and the number of people repatriated was low,[68] as Table 11 below shows.[69] Just what 'fit for work' meant was not clearly spelled out, but one doctor commented that if the same standard of fitness were to be applied as that for military recruits in Germany, only one quarter to one third of the recruits would be deemed fit.

Table 11
Repatriated labourers 1905–1913

Year	Total	Repatriated	Per cent
1905	2763	15	0.54
1906	n/a		
1907	2865	59	2.05
1908	4554	158	3.46
1909	4125	107	2.59
1910	6428	94	1.46
1911	7704	34	0.44
1912	8245	66	0.80
1913	10848	150	1.38

Smallpox

While the introduction of dysentery had probably been unavoidable, this was not so with smallpox. Its introduction to Kaiser-Wilhelmsland on the Norddeutscher Lloyd steamer *Lübeck,* which arrived in Friedrich-Wilhelmshafen on 1 June 1893,[70] was a major calamity. Quarantine legis-lation[71]—mentioning specifically cholera, yellow fever, plague, smallpox,

68 Casual day labourers did not undergo medical examination. MB 1906/7: 195-6.
69 Compiled from *Amtsblatt* and Annual Reports
70 Smallpox was introduced by a Malay child according to *NKWL*, a Malay stoker on board the *Lübeck* according to the Annual Report. It is likely that more than one infected person was on board ship.
71 Quarantäne Ordnung für das Schutzgebiet der Neuguinea Kompagnie, 29 September 1891. *DKG* 1: 518-22

measles, scarlet fever, typhoid fever—failed its first serious test. The legislation was enacted in 1891 following an outbreak of cholera on a labour transport from Singapore and Surabaya in November 1890, from which the infection was transmitted to labourers on Hatzfeldhafen station, where twenty-eight succumbed before it could be contained.[72] If authorities believed that legislation would prove a shield against infectious diseases, they were quickly proved wrong. At best it gave the impression that preventive measures were taken. There was no legislation to enforce vaccination of all labourers coming from Asia, surely the crucial measure to prevent the introduction of smallpox. General vaccination was introduced only after the outbreak of the epidemic.[73] Yet the cholera epidemic should have alerted the administration to the ease with which an infectious or contagious disease could be introduced, and the need to make use of all preventive measures available.

Quarantine requirements were flouted when smallpox suspects were on the *Lübeck*. Against the advice of Dr Frobenius[74] and without his knowledge, Chinese and Javanese coolies and their families were put ashore and transferred from Friedrich-Wilhelmshafen to Stephansort, the plantation centre with a large Melanesian labour force. There new smallpox cases—mainly children—were isolated, but not the full contingent of people from the *Lübeck*. The first Melanesian smallpox patient, a man from Mioko whose young child had come down with the infection, was hospitalised on 25 June 1893.[75]

The recommendation by Frobenius that the company vessel *Ysabel* be sent urgently to Australia to fetch good fresh lymph was met with delaying tactics.[76] The main stumbling block was cost, estimated at around 9,000 Mark and the risk to the ship of a trip south.[77] The company management was confronted with an unprecedented situation, one that no one in Berlin had ever imagined in their wildest fantasies about New Guinea and, when weighing costs and possible risks to company property against public health, the company's financial interests prevailed.

---

72   *NKWL* 1891: 13
73   RKA 2428:50
74   Doctor with the Rhenish Mission from 1890–1900
75   Frobenius letter in *Berichte der Rheinischen Missionsgesellschaft*, 1893: 338-9
76   Frobenius letter. Present at the meeting were Schmiele, Administrator of the NGC, von Hagen, Administrator of the Astrolabe Company, Captain Dallmann of the *Ysabel*, Drs Jentzsch and Frobenius.
77   The company had lost the steamer *Ottilie* the year before. *NKWL* 1892: 40

The epidemic quickly spread to the labourers in Stephansort, Erima and Constantinhafen; from there to native villages, to Maraga and finally to Yomba plantation by November. Lymph arrived by the beginning of July from the State Vaccination Institute in Batavia;[78] a month had elapsed before vaccination could begin, long enough to ensure the spread of the infection. No Europeans became infected—vaccination being compulsory in Germany since 1875 under the Imperial Vaccination Act of 1874.[79]

There is another aspect to the sorry smallpox story: the new General Manager of the Astrolabe Company, von Hagen, was on board the *Lübeck,* as was the new company doctor, Jentzsch. It is inconceivable that neither of them knew of the outbreak on board ship. Their disregard of basic quarantine measures was, to say the least, a serious neglect of duties.

Despite the vaccination program, sporadic outbreaks of smallpox continued among labourers on the company's plantations and it was not until May 1894 that it was believed to have been successfully eradicated in the Astrolabe Bay region, nearly a year after the outbreak. But infection lingered on for at least another two years when a newly arrived labour recruit from Rook Island brought smallpox with him to Friedrich-Wilhelmshafen in 1896. Another 17 labourers contracted the infection before this last flare-up could be brought under control.[80] As far as could be established, smallpox had spread widely among the population in the hinterland of the station, and along the Huon Gulf. It also spread to the north coast of New Britain as far east as the Nakanai district and the Witu Islands. However, quarantine measures, together with sufficient time to vaccinate, prevented a spread to the most densely populated region of the colony, the Gazelle Peninsula.

There was speculation whether there had been earlier smallpox epidemics in Kaiser-Wilhelmsland. The company, perhaps trying to put forward mitigating circumstances, suggested that a smallpox epidemic had occurred among natives seven years earlier.[81] Dr Hagen, who arrived during a renewed flare-up, argued that the prompt and powerful reactions of Melanesians to vaccination demonstrated that people had no immunity whatsoever and he regarded this as clear proof that smallpox was new to the country.[82]

There were no further smallpox outbreaks after 1896. The epidemic in the 1890s had left behind a deep fear; quarantine restrictions were enforced strictly

78 AR 1891-93: 81
79 C. Huerkamp, 'The History of Smallpox Vaccination in Germany,' *JCH* 20 (1985): 617-35
80 NKWL 1896: 24
81 *NKWL* 1894: 24
82 Hagen 41

and vaccination was compulsory for all recruits, despite the reluctance of some employers to have them vaccinated because this often resulted in a secondary infection, so that a man could not work for some time.[83] People living within reach of the government or of missions were also vaccinated. The smallpox epidemic in Sydney early in 1914 caused no small panic in Rabaul; everybody in the district was vaccinated or revaccinated,[84] with the result that at the outbreak of war, when doctors decided to use up all stocks of lymph, it was very difficult to find any unvaccinated people in the district.[85]

Malaria

After the turn of the century, when malaria prophylaxis was officially part of the public health program, malaria declined but did not disappear, and doctors had to explore why improvements in health fell short of expectations.

In the Bismarck Archipelago the number of patients in government hospitals because of malaria from 1902 on ranged between 10 and 20 per cent of all patients (see Appendix VII for morbidity in government native hospitals in Herbertshöhe and Rabaul). Malaria screening of all servants and their children in European households and plantation labourers living close to a residence were carried out by Dr Dempwolff in 1902,[86] and confirmed Koch's theory that children and people from malaria-free regions were prime carriers of malaria parasites. These test results were sent to each employer together with instructions on when and how quinine had to be administered.[87] But, as Wendland reported, "most Europeans had neither the patience nor the energy" to enforce the program.

The quininisation program remained a constant source of frustration for doctors. Not because labourers refused to take quinine: on the contrary, doctors repeatedly commented that native people had no objection to taking it, quite unlike Europeans. Small planters, whose labourers were infected, refused quinine prophylaxis as it apparently reduced the labourers' capacity to work. The laudable exception was the Catholic Mission; the Brother in charge of the sick ward undertook the work "with great understanding and zeal"; if people there could not be convinced of the

83 Wendland in Denkschrift, Anlage Aktenstück 54: 397, *Stenographische Berichte der Verhandlungen des Reichstags*, 1903/04 (11. Legislaturperiode, 2. Session) 1. Anlegeband

84 RKA 5773: 108

85 Kersten to Wick 24.8.1914, G255/807

86 Dempwolff, 'Malaria-Expedition': 81–132

87 Archival file Robert-Koch-Institut

necessity for quinine, it could be enforced with a "certain compulsion".[88]

Even among police troops and labourers working for the government systematic quinine intake proved possible only for those permanently based in Herbertshöhe. As long as a doctor supervised the intake, prophylaxis worked quite well, but sizeable numbers of police troops were absent for lengthy periods; during such absence, dispensing of quinine was neglected and among the returning troops were large numbers of newly infected malaria patients. Even when a program was started before the onset of the rainy period, it could not be completed if troops were suddenly dispatched elsewhere. Men in the land survey team were not given quinine during their absence from Herbertshöhe. As the surveyor in charge of the team neglected to take quinine himself, it was unrealistic to expect him to hand it out to his workers. For men working on road construction and labourers on plantations away from Herbertshöhe, the situation was similar—local managers showed "insufficient interest" in malaria prevention.[89] Extensive clearing work in Simpsonhafen created new breeding grounds for mosquitoes and contributed a great deal to an increase of malaria. The program carried out by Sister Hertzer in villages along Blanche Bay and among construction workers of the Norddeutscher Lloyd proved of benefit to Melanesians, and reduced but did not prevent malaria among Chinese artisans.[90] But new artisans arrived in the colony regularly; police troopers with their families were brought in from the Caroline Islands, and all were highly susceptible to malaria; prisoners brought to Herbertshöhe became infected and had to be treated to prevent their carrying malaria home to an uninfected area.[91] New arrivals were therefore the majority of malaria patients at the hospital.

On the basis of her experience, and less despondent than doctors, Sister Hertzer submitted a proposal for a comprehensive long-term program to protect all people on the Gazelle Peninsula against malaria. She suggested that a number of paramedical staff be employed, each one responsible for a small section of the Gazelle Peninsula, to work on malaria therapy and prophylaxis, as well as the general education of the population.[92] Hertzer's proposals

88 Wendland in Denkschrift, Anlage Aktenstück 54: 395, *Stenographische Berichte der Verhandlungen des Reichstags,* 1903/04 (11. Legislaturperiode, 2. Session) 1. Anlegeband
89 MB 1903/04: 182-7
90 Hertzer reports 30 September 1903, 31 December 1903, 31 March 1904. Archives Robert-Koch-Institut
91 MB 1903/04: 183-5
92 Hertzer report 31 March 1904

came to nothing "as Treasury had advised that 1905 budgets were extremely tight and economies had to be made everywhere".[93]

Wendland, increasingly sceptical about eliminating malaria, proposed that new housing for colonists should be built well away from labourers' barracks. In his view the newcomers built their houses and the accommodation for their labourers and domestic staff too close together, a proximity which created a serious health threat to settlers.[94] When it came to planning the new capital, Rabaul, the call for segregation was taken up by Dr Seibert on the same grounds.

Action on other recommended measures, such as the destruction of mosquito breeding grounds by filling in trenches and swampy ground, was very slow. Yet, when badly designed irrigation trenches on a Forsayth plantation were filled in after years of repeated requests by Wendland, this work was credited with greatly reducing malaria among labourers in the district,[95] as was infilling around Vunapope.[96]

Dysentery

Dysentery was first reported in the Gazelle Peninsula when a group of labourers returned from Queensland in the early 1880s. It remained endemic, with frequent epidemics in the labour force. During 1896/97 fifteen out of thirty-three deaths were due to dysentery, as were most deaths in the second half of 1899, and again in 1901.[97] A reduction in the incidence during 1902 was reflected in a drop in the mortality rate: one in five deaths were due to dysentery compared with close to half in 1896/97.[98]

Dr Danneil suspected water as the source of infection and recommended that, while rainwater tanks had to be relied on as the topography of Herbertshöhe did not lend itself to the construction of wells, they had to be carefully maintained. Labourers should be given sufficient quantities of lightly sweetened tea during dysentery epidemics so as to avoid further infection through dirty tank water.[99]

Judging by the frequent epidemics among labourers in the district, these

---

93   Internal memorandum Colonial Department, 16.6.1904. RKA 5769: 67-8
94   Wendland report in Denkschrift, Anlage Aktenstück 54, *Stenographische Berichte der Verhandlungen des Reichstags,* 1903/04 (11. Legislaturperiode, 2. Session) 1. Anlegeband
95   RKA 5772: 4 ff
96   MB 1903/04: 187
97   NKWL 1898: 32-33; Aktenstück 437: 3096, *Stenographische Berichte der Verhandlungen des Reichstags,* 1900/02 (10. Legislaturperiode, 2. Session) 5. Anlegeband
98   AR NGC 1902/03: 20-21, RKA 2420: 8 ff
99   *NKWL* 1898: 35-6

recommendations met with indifference. The foundation years of Rabaul illustrate the slowness with which basic facilities were introduced; Dr Seibert's efforts to get the government to provide basic sanitary facilities have been discussed in the first chapter. Doctors who followed him stressed the urgent need for unpolluted water and sanitary facilities, adding that the barracks also badly needed improvements.[100] Meanwhile, epidemics recurred regularly and dysentery deaths multiplied, with up to one third of dysentery patients perishing. An epidemic which began in Rabaul in 1906 spread throughout the Gazelle Peninsula and affected the whole population over the next six months, with a repetition in the following year. Of the forty-nine dysentery patients in 1906 at the Herbertshöhe hospital, fifteen died, and in the following year so did eleven of the twenty-four patients.[101]

The government recognised that problems were due to the lack of clean water and sanitary facilities but, until a decision was made in Berlin whether Rabaul should become the capital of the colony, no capital works were undertaken; the hospital and barracks were temporary only, and sanitation was ignored altogether. When it was decided to move the seat of government to Rabaul, the construction of permanent buildings and sanitary facilities began, more than ten years after the attention of the authorities was first drawn to the problem, while all the time the population of Rabaul increased and dysentery did not diminish.

In mid-1909 new barracks were ready in the new Melanesian quarter of Rabaul and houses had been built in the Malay quarter. Pit latrines were installed and, while awaiting the construction of wells in all quarters of Rabaul, rain water was stored in tanks. The results were remarkable: dysentery outbreaks among labourers and police in the new quarters ceased,[102] and in later years remained confined to sporadic cases. With the construction of wells in the various quarters in Rabaul, a good water supply was ensured and health conditions had become satisfactory.[103] Living in barracks was an opportunity for soldiers and labourers to learn the principles of personal hygiene, with stiff penalties for non-compliance.[104]

The provisions that the government made for its troops and labour force

100 For example, Wendland, 20 September 1906, RKA 5730: 144 ff; Born in July 1908, RKA 5771: 45 ff; Wick in March 1909, RKA 3774: 59 ff
101 MB 1906/07: 204; 221; 1907/08: 416; 439
102 Wick, quarterly report 1.7.-30.6.1909, RKA 5771: 186 ff
103 Wick, quarterly report 1.4.-30.6.1910, RKA 5772: 10 ff
104 Soldier Butsitli was fined 1 Mark, the wages for the whole of June 1909, for soiling the latrines. G255/743

were indeed exemplary. Unfortunately no one seemed to be willing to emulate these achievements. Dysentery epidemics recurred on plantations throughout the Peninsula. As employers neither took immediate measures for isolation and disinfection, nor sent patients to hospital when the first symptoms appeared, an attempt was made to educate employers on the nature of dysentery and its treatment and prevention.[105] Continuing outbreaks suggest that the advice was ignored; yet no steps were taken by the government to compel employers to provide elementary facilities. It remained a matter of managing an epidemic and bringing it under temporary control, rather than preventing it. Death rates for dysentery patients remained high, especially if there was concurrent illness such as malaria, lung disease or extended ulcerations.[106] In the plantation hospitals of the New Guinea Company and Forsayth & Company at least one third of all deaths were due to dysentery. For example, in 1909 of 122 deaths in the three company hospitals, forty-four were due to dysentery. The last period for which records are available still showed the same pattern: twenty-one of the sixty-three dysentery cases died in the first quarter of 1914.[107] Not much had changed on plantations since Dr Seibert pointed out that the Reich was spending millions each year for research on tropical diseases, and training and equipping doctors to work in the colonies as public health officers, but that in practice their advice was largely ignored, with the result that appalling sanitary conditions persisted.[108]

Convicts were probably at the greatest risk of dysentery and other diarrhoeal diseases. The first indication that sanitary conditions in the gaol were inadequate came in 1902, when of the eight dysentery deaths four were convicts.[109] Poor accommodation, lack of sanitation, and meagre food rations, created shocking conditions.[110] Convicts had to empty and clean toilet buckets in European houses and the hospitals, a job that exposed them to faecal matter, with no opportunity to wash properly afterwards.[111] Improvements to prison conditions in Rabaul were not made until 1908, when accommodation and sanitation were bettered and each convict was issued with soap and individual eating utensils.[112] Conditions remained appalling in other prisons.

105 *Amtsblatt* 1909: 51-4, an article by Wick in which he described dysentery symptoms and immediate actions to be taken, like isolation of patient, castor oil, and sweetened tea.
106 RKA 5772: 223
107 MB 1909/10: 475. Kersten, report 1.1.-31.3.1914. RKA 5773: 106
108 Seibert to governor, 9.9.1906, RKA 5730: 138
109 Wendland, report in Denkschrift, Anlage Aktenstück 54: 396, *Stenographische Berichte der Verhandlungen des Reichstags,* 1903/04 (11. Legislaturperiode, 2. Session) 1. Anlegeband
110 MB 1906/07: 203-4
111 Wendland, report 1.10.-31.12.1908, RKA 5771: 82 ff
112 MB 1907/08: 415-6

The poor conditions of Herbertshöhe gaol made it virtually impossible to eradicate dysentery.[113] In Namatanai the small, low, unhygienic, corrugated iron covered shed which served as a gaol, was a "much harder punishment than most convicts deserved".[114] While conditions of government facilities in Rabaul were being improved, on other stations progress was slower and gaols had low priority.

There was one notable exception to the dysentery saga. Following an epidemic on Matupi in January 1909, Father Bögershausen from the Sacred Heart Mission joined forces with the doctor to combat dysentery on the island. Constant exhortation to cleanliness, supervision of all housing and enforced clearing of the surroundings meant that during 1909 there was not a single case of dysentery on Matupi despite another outbreak in Rabaul in April.[115]

Cause of death in native hospitals on the Gazelle Peninsula for the years 1902 to 1911 was listed in 790 cases. Of these, 254, a fraction under one third, were due to dysentery. The figures suggest that there was plenty of room for sanitary improvements.

While the focus on the discussion has been on the Gazelle Peninsula, dysentery problems were similar in other centres. In Kaewieng, where only sporadic cases were reported in the first few years,[116] the situation deteriorated and, as the number of labourers increased, so did the incidence of dysentery.[117] Sanitary improvements put an end to severe epidemics, but dysentery remained a constant threat. In Namatanai there was an outbreak of dysentery on Bopire, a newly established plantation of the Bismarck Archipelago Gesellschaft, while Dr Born was in the district. His quick action soon brought it under control, but left him wondering how the incompetent medical orderly was going to cope with other outbreaks.[118] In Friedrich-Wilhelmshafen the situation was somewhat different. While dysentery was endemic, epidemics occurred far less frequently than in the Bismarck Archipelago. Arrangements for sanitary waste disposal differed from those in the Bismarck Archipelago, small huts being built over the water minimising contact with faecal matter. Nevertheless, there was a serious bacillary dysentery epidemic in Friedrich-Wilhelmshafen in 1912 with nineteen deaths.[119]

Discussion has centred on labourers who were working near enough to a

113 MB 1906/07: 203-4
114 Born, report 29.7.1908, RKA 2311: 56
115 MB 1909/10: 487
116 MB 1904/05: 202
117 MB 1905/06: 287-9
118 Report 29.7.1908, RKA 2311: 55 ff
119 MB 1912/13: 52

medical service to be brought to a doctor. As new plantations were set up remote from European centres, increasing numbers of labourers worked in areas where doctors' visits were rare. For example, at the Bopire plantation in central New Ireland, the company employed an untrained German medical orderly. What little experience he may have had did not prepare him for any of the work to be done in a plantation hospital, so that Dr Born insisted that the man be sent to the Namatanai hospital to learn a few basic skills.[120]

To ensure minimum standards for labourers, the 1909 Labour Ordinance prescribed government supervision of working conditions, in particular accommodation, rations, health care and wages.[121] Supervision may well have been effective in districts where government officials were able to carry out regular inspections. There is some doubt about its effect in remote districts. While Dr Kopp was on Manus in 1912 to bring a dysentery epidemic under control, he also inspected all establishments. On the Wahlen plantation on Maron (Western Islands), everything was in order in the plantation hospital. Basic surgical tools for first aid were well cared for and there was a good supply of medications for the most common ailments. On the Hernsheim and Komine plantations he found the very opposite. Accommodation for patients in simple bush huts was most primitive, and surgical tools were non-existent or unusable. The medicine chests contained only a few patent medications—Chlorodyne and Painkiller on the Hernsheim plantations, Chinese and Japanese panaceas on the Komine plantations. Not one person on these plantations had heard about regulations regarding domestic dispensaries.[122]

Kopp's inspection highlighted the difficulties the government had in enforcing its ruling on medical care, and in general, to ensure that labour conditions in remote districts were upheld by employers. Inspections in such regions depended on the availability of staff and transport; doctors were busy at their local hospital; what time they had for inspection tours had to fit in with shipping schedules. There is no information to indicate how frequent inspection tours were, or how effective policing was, and little is known on how the labour force fared on remote plantations.

---

120 Born, report 29.7.1908, RKA 2311: 57
121 Paragraph 13, Verordnung des Gouverneurs von Deutsch-Neuguinea betreffend Anwerbung und Ausführung von Eingeborenen im Schutzgebiet Deutsch-Neuguinea. 4 March 1909. *DKG* 13: 147-53
122 Hahl to Colonial Office, 23.7.1912, RKA 5952: 98

Nutrition

The change from a traditional diet to one based on polished rice was fatal to many labourers. It was a change imposed by plantation companies who found it more convenient and cheaper to import rice, rather than diverting a section of the labour force, and of land, to growing local foods.

The New Guinea Company made much of the importance of good food for labourers and its effort to provide it. In the Recruitment Ordinance of 15 August 1888,[123] required rations for labourers were 500 grams of rice and 1.5 kilograms of root crops daily plus 750 grams of meat or fish per week. The rice ration was replaceable with root crops or bread. The same rations were applicable for labour depots[124] and by implication were the guide for labourers on plantations. The same provisions were made in the 1901 Labour Ordinance.[125]

Legal provisions were one thing, their implementation another matter, and the company increasingly failed to follow its own prescription. When the company began planting operations, and the labour force was small, a certain amount of food was grown on the stations. Maize was often planted as a first crop to prepare the ground for main plantings, and root crops were planted as catch-crops in cotton plantings. Harvests varied a great deal from satisfactory to failures because of droughts or wet weather, or destruction by wild pigs. Yams were soon found to be too demanding in labour to be worth the effort of planting.[126] It seems, however, that in the early days, depending on the season, sufficient food crops were grown to supplement rice, the staple food, so there was some variety and reasonable nutrition.

This changed with the move from Finschhafen to Friedrich-Wilhelmshafen where, ostensibly to avoid the danger of miasmas developing when the ground was first dug, no food crops were planted. With missionary Bergmann as intermediary, trade with local natives was established which ensured a supply of root crops.[127] However, not enough food was produced to supply the ever increasing number of labourers—the local population was too small to

---

123 Verordnung des Landeshauptmanns, betr. die Anwerbung und Ausführung von Eingeborenen als Arbeiter, 15 August 1888, *DKG* 1: 535
124 Verordnung des Landeshauptmanns betr. Arbeiterdepots im Schutzgebiet der Neuguinea Kompagnie, 16 August 1888, *DKG* 1: 549
125 Verordnung des Gouverneurs von Deutsch-Neuguinea, betr. die Ausführung und Anwerbung von Eingeborenen als Arbeiter in Deutsch Neuguinea, 31.7.1901. *DKG* 6: 363
126 *NKWL* 1888: 150; 1890: 12; 68-69
127 *NKWL* 1892: 25

produce the amount of food required and, more importantly in the company's view, lacked the incentive to do so, as it did not have enough wants to encourage large scale production for the purpose of marketing and trading.[128] On Erima station the only food available for labourers was rice, and meat was not supplied for months.[129] In Constantinhafen the staple was also rice, with an occasional supplement of bananas or root crops;[130] food shortages were not uncommon and Kaiser-Wilhelmsland came into disrepute not only because of death and disease, but also because of lack of food.[131]

Reports of harvests of 20,000 kilograms of sweet potatoes over a period of six months[132] may sound impressive, yet if the approximately one hundred and fifty labourers on the station during that period[133] were issued with the stipulated rations of 1.5 kilograms of root crops, this harvest was only eighty-eight days supply and more than twice the amount was needed for the six months' period, in addition to 75 kilograms of rice per day and the weekly issues of fish or meat. In Constantinhafen, with about one hundred and seventy-five labourers, 250 kilograms of green maize were used per day during June 1892.[134] Clearly, large quantities of food had to be grown to meet the daily needs for any length of time, and not even imports from Bismarck Archipelago could meet demand.[135]

Increasing reliance on polished rice as staple food unavoidably led to beriberi, and the first report dates from the second half of 1890 in Finschhafen, with a steady increase in the incidence which reached large proportions in Stephansort in 1893, if not earlier. It was widespread among coolies and increasingly also affected Melanesians who, it was believed, had been infected by the former. It was readily preventable by supplying labourers with their accustomed diet; instead, for nearly twenty years doctors in German New Guinea searched for remedies and a scientific explanation for the causes of beriberi.

To deal with beriberi the company hired a medical practitioner, Dr Hagen, who had had thirteen years' experience on tobacco plantations on Sumatra. There he had had ample opportunity to observe beriberi patients and he had noted a number of social conditions which caused beriberi, and for which he sought

128 Rose report 30.6.1892, RKA 6512: 51ff
129 Kindt, manager of Erima station, to Reich Chancellor 2.9.1891, RKA 2410: 327ff.
130 NKWL 1892: 27
131 Rose to AA 19.11.1891, RKA 2302: 37 f; von Bennigsen to AA 23.6.1900, RKA 2307: 61

132 Harvest in Finschhafen from May to October 1889. NKWL 1890:10
133 NKWL 1890: 12
134 NKWL 1893:22
135 50 tons of yam were exported from the Gazelle Peninsula to KWL early in 1892, RKA 6512: 77

a medical remedy: nearly without exception beriberi affected people on whom certain restraints were imposed in relation to housing, food or work. He had observed the disease almost exclusively in prisons, in hospitals, on hulks, and on tobacco plantations. Living in small cramped quarters, where each occupant had just enough room to sleep, favoured in his view the outbreak and the spread of the disease. Only very rarely had he seen free and independent people suffering from it. In addition to the social conditions which ostensibly gave rise to beriberi, Hagen also found it to be a disease that was race and gender specific. Chinese and Javanese were most prone to it, and usually suffered it in its hydropic form. Next came Malays who for the most part suffered from atrophic beriberi. It was very rare among Tamils (in the Dutch East Indies) and Europeans; men were much more likely to be affected than women. Yet there was little he could do for these patients. Only when "unfit" coolies and those recovering from beriberi were repatriated—a "radical and courageous" decision taken on the advice of the resident doctor—did death rates begin to fall.

Hagen was sure that the change in diet of the native labourers on taking up work on a plantation had a detrimental effect which manifested itself in various gastro-enteric diseases and he therefore condemned the company's failure to establish plantations for staple foods. The company had resorted to the quick and easy rice, on the basis that "rice [was] the staple food in the tropics for half of mankind". In Hagen's view it was essential for labourers to be provided with the range of foods to which they were accustomed since childhood so that they could acclimatise to the new surroundings without too many difficulties.[136] The irony is that Hagen did not know how right he was when he advocated a traditional diet.

Poor nutrition was not restricted to plantations, for doctors noted that some patients suddenly developed beriberi symptoms after four to six weeks in hospital, especially during the wet season, and died because of complications, such as dysentery.[137] In gaols beriberi was not uncommon.[138]

The first cases of beriberi in the Herbertshöhe hospital were Melanesian labourers who had been sent there from Kaiser-Wilhelmsland in the hope that "a change of air" would help them to recuperate. Most recovered quickly without medical intervention.[139] Other beriberi cases hospitalised there were

136 Hagen 35, 39, 47
137 Wendland 'Beri-Beri' 237-44; MB 1905/6: 291
138 Runge, report 16.5.1908, RKA 2311: 79-80
139 MB 1905/06: 290

from ships' crews. As many were Chinese, and one or two Melanesians usually fell sick, the myth of infection through Chinese was perpetuated. The absence of beriberi on plantations in the Bismarck Archipelago was explained by the fact that no Chinese were on plantations,[140] but after 1904, when beriberi became widespread in the Gazelle Peninsula and also in Kaewieng, that explanation no longer held. With the expansion of colonial activities, the disease pattern well known in Kaiser-Wilhelmsland—malaria, dysentery and beriberi—was repeated in the Bismarck Archipelago, and beriberi spread to all occupational groups: seamen, police troops, plantation labourers and labour convicts. The food supply was also a repetition of the Kaiser-Wilhelmsland experience: in the early days demand for staple crops had stimulated production and local people had enlarged their plantations,[141] but with the growth in the labour force, food requirements could no longer be met locally. Dependency on rice grew and it increasingly became the staple on Gazelle Peninsula plantations as well as in other districts; the only variation being a pig or some other food that labourers managed to steal or trade.[142]

As the number of beriberi patients grew, so did the number of theories on its causes and cures. Doctors experimented with diets, as they knew that a connection had been made between diet and beriberi. Hagen's prescription of "strong broth" to replace rice and dried fish brought no results and he dismissed the theory.[143] When Dr Hoffmann arrived in Friedrich-Wilhelmshafen, he prescribed a change from polished rice to cured rice, the method developed in the Dutch East Indies for the treatment of beriberi. He was sceptical that the rapid recovery he observed in many cases was due to the diet, but it was "easy, cheap and certainly not harmful".[144] While working in Friedrich-Wilhelmshafen in 1906, Runge noted that there was a definite improvement in their condition, when the diet of beriberi patients consisted mainly of yams, taro, fish and coconut and very little rice. When such supplies ran out due to seasonal factors, and rice was again the staple food, their recovery came to a standstill.[145]

An outbreak among road construction labourers in Kabakada convinced Wendland that the theory of an unidentified poisonous substance developing in cooked rice stored for some hours was correct. Labourers worked an extremely hard 10-hour day under punishing conditions, exposed to the sun. Taro, yams and sweet potatoes were unobtainable in sufficient quantities and

140 MB 1903/04: 188
141 Rose report 20.6.1892, RKA 6512: 51 ff
142 Kolbe to Government, RKA 2311: 43 ff
143 Hagen 50
144 MB 1903/04: 235
145 MB 1906/07: 227

each man was given the standard food ration of 600 grams of rice per day and once a week a one pound tin of meat. Many saved part of the rice cooked in the evening and ate it next morning, after a poison had developed during overnight storage. Further confirmation of the theory was the fact that local people who worked on the road provided their own food and remained free of beriberi.[146] His recommendation for sweet tea and ship's biscuits in a mid-morning break was rejected by the Governor.[147] Beriberi outbreaks among these labourers stopped as soon as road work was completed and they returned to Herbertshöhe.

In Kaewieng Runge decided to test the diet theory by sending all beriberi patients to a small island in the Nusa Waters, where they were accommodated in huts built in the traditional style, and were issued with rice and meat rations and given tobacco to trade for local food. All recovered quickly. Even this result did not convince Runge and he suggested that psychological causes, such as living in the traditional style, contributed as much to the improvement as a change in diet.[148]

In the same year experiments began in the Rabaul Botanical Garden with growing mung beans—*phaseolus aureus*[149] or *katjang idjoe* bean as the Germans called it, adopting the Malay name—following reports from the Dutch East Indies that their addition had proved successful in the cure and prevention of beriberi.[150] It took another year or two to convince all doctors that nutrition was the crucial factor and that mung beans were effective as a cure and prophylactic for beriberi. By 1911 all hospital patients were given around 150 grams of mung beans per day, a quantity which proved curative as well as preventive. The beans were cooked together with rice to ensure that the unknown agent which affected beriberi was not lost in cooking water.[151] As thiamine is a water soluble vitamin, it was a stroke of luck that the beans were cooked in this way. After these experimentations there was no longer any need for beriberi isolation wards, which were attached to all hospitals, as beriberi was clearly not infectious. The next step was to convince plantation and shipping owners that mung beans should become part of the everyday diet of all labourers.

A veritable mung bean campaign was begun by government authorities. The Government Gazette carried articles on the prevention and cure of

146 MB 1907/08: 424-6
147 RKA 5769: 178
148 MB 1909/10: 489-94

149 Professor James J. Fox drew my attention to the change in botanic nomenclature. At the time mung bean was classified as *P. radiatus*.
150 MB 1909/10: 489-94
151 MB 1911/12: 498

beriberi and the Botanical Garden regularly made bean seeds available free of charge to employers.[152] Pupils at the government school were taught to grow mung beans in the school garden.[153] The zealous promotion of mung beans had reached a point of absurdity; mung beans after all only corrected a nutritional deficiency unknown in a traditional diet.

While a diet of cured rice and mung beans cured patients and also prevented hospital beriberi, there was no sudden halt in the incidence elsewhere. Not only did beriberi persist on the ships of the Norddeutscher Lloyd and on small vessels, it also recurred on plantations. Planters were not readily convinced that a varied diet was essential and it was only at the beginning of 1914 that a decrease of beriberi cases during the wet season was noted in the Rabaul district.[154] Away from the main centre the necessary changes had not been introduced, and there was one more severe epidemic on a plantation while German doctors were in New Guinea. In Hernsheim plantations in New Ireland, with a large number of recruits from the St. Matthias Group (in the north of the Bismarck Archipelago), seventy-eight cases occurred from August to November 1914. At the doctor's insistence the diet of patients was changed to fresh fish and fresh fruit (pawpaw, pineapple and melons), and as a substitute for rice *saksak*, a mixture of sago and grated coconuts. The results were so striking that the doctor convinced the plantation management to change the diet of all labourers.[155]

In their response doctors epitomised medical reactions to beriberi problems. The notion that a bacterial agent was the cause of the disease so dominated thinking that, for most of them, the idea that the absence of a substance was the cause was contrary to anything they knew and therefore hard to accept. Eventually empirical evidence was so strong that dietary changes were advocated and implemented in a clinical situation before the actual substance, thiamine or Vitamin B1, was discovered in 1911 by the medical scientist Casimir Funk.[156] The next step in New Guinea, convincing plantation owners of the efficacy of a varied diet, was as slow and difficult as it had been to convince doctors that it was absence, not presence, of a substance that caused beriberi.

The provision of food was a highly contentious question, viewed from different angles by planters and administration. For planters rations were an expense that ate into profits and therefore had to be kept low. The first con-

152 *Amtsblatt* 1910:62; 1911:116
153 Draft AR 1913/14: 161
154 Kersten, quarterly report 1.1.-31.3.1914, RKA 5773: 106

155 Dieterlen, 'Ueber eine im Jahre 1914 in der Südsee beobachtete Beriberi-Epidemie,' *ASTH* 20 (1916): 306-11
156 Machlin, L.J., ed., *Handbook of Vitamins* (New York, Dekker, 1984) 247

frontation between the two parties began in 1898, when Hahl attempted to protect fishing and breeding grounds by banning fishing with dynamite in the waters of Blanche Bay and the Duke of York islands[157] which had become seriously depleted. A total ban for the whole colony was issued in 1904[158] and, as could be expected, was strongly attacked by plantation companies, as this denied them access to cheap and nutritious food relished by labourers. A proposal by Hahl to fish with nets was dismissed as unrealistic under prevailing conditions.[159] The New Guinea Company exerted enough pressure so that over the next two years exemptions to the ban were introduced.[160] Another attempt to protect fishing grounds was made in 1913, when a prohibition on fishing with dynamite was issued to take effect on 1 January 1914.[161]

The ban on fishing was a step not taken lightly by Hahl. He was aware of the importance of fish as a source of food but, confronted with the exploitation and rapid destruction of a valuable resource, he sought to protect it. The planters took a very short term view and were concerned only with the immediate cost of rations, whereas Hahl wanted to husband these resources to ensure a long term food supply.

Another confrontation began when doctors came to see sound nutrition as a chief weapon in the fight against disease. They kept up to date with nutritional research which initially was carried out to investigate the nutritional requirements of Europeans in the tropics,[162] and then was extended to assess the requirements of native workers.[163] Armed with this knowledge doctors increasingly related the generally unsatisfactory state of health among labourers to inadequate nutrition. Lack of resistance to dysentery and pneumonia in particular were directly attributed to undernutrition, so clearly visible in the "famished look" of many labourers.[164] Many men were hospitalised simply

---

157 Verordnung des Landeshauptmanns, betr. das Verbot des Fischens mit Dynamit, 2 Dec. 1898; *DKG* 3: 167; NGC to AA 3.2.1899, RKA 7651: 3 ff

158 Verordnung des Gouverneurs, betr. das Verbot des Fischens unter Anwendung von Sprengstoffen, 1 Dec. 1904. *DKG* 8: 257-8

159 NGK to AA 3.5.1905, RKA 7651: 14

160 Ordinances of 13 Dec. 1905, 16 March 1906 and 11 Dec. 1906. *DKG* 9: 278; *DKG* 9: 140; *DKG* 10: 345

161 Bekanntmachung Gouverneur betr. das Verbot des Fischeschiessens, 17 April 1913. *DKB* 1913: 577

162 See for instance Ranke, *Ueber die Einwirkung des Tropenklimas auf die Ernährung des Menschen* (Berlin, 1900)

163 A path-breaking study was carried out in the Dutch East Indies in 1897 in order to regulate the nutrition of native convicts. See C.L. van der Burg, L'alimentation des Européens et des travailleurs indigènes aux pays chauds. *Janus* 10 (1905): 88-94

164 Born, report to Hahl, 25.10.1909, RKA 2311: 202

because of malnutrition, evidence that legislative guidelines were ignored. Each company provided rations that it considered appropriate, even if this meant poor quality salt meat of which little was edible, or dried fish spoilt during storage, so that it was a danger to health.[165] Legal prescriptions were needed to ensure proper nutrition. Proposals for increased rations came up against the intransigence of planters. Forsayth & Company, for example, submitted that under existing regulations food cost per labourer per year was 96 Mark. The proposed rations would cost 124 Mark per year, a substantial cost increase of around 37500 Mark for the 1340 labourers employed by the company. The Bismarck Archipelago Gesellschaft estimated its cost increase for its 400 labourers at around 14400 Mark.[166] In a compromise, daily rations were fixed at 625 grams of rice or 3 kg of root crops plus 750 grams of meat or fish, with a rider that these rations were calculated for a body weight of 60 kg and that rations had to be increased depending on a labourer's physique.[167]

The discussion of the 1909 labour ordinance occurred at a time when scientific research had provided doctors with enough ammunition to argue about calorific values of food; but there was no scientific proof of the importance of nutritional content. What was known was the amount of calories needed to provide a labourer with enough energy to work, and the discussion centred around the minimum numbers of calories needed to ensure maximum work. Planters would not supply workers with more calories than absolutely needed. Therefore, when the new ordinance was adopted, rations were fixed at an amount commensurate with minimum calorific requirements, but they were nutritionally poorer than before. The provision of rice or root crops ensured that planters relied on rice. As little as a year later there was enough evidence from government hospitals that beriberi was curable and preventable with a sound diet.

A new labour ordinance was drafted at the end of 1913 which again detailed rations. The latest advances in nutritional research and regard to traditional food of labourers formed the basis of the recommendations. Rice was to be reduced to 300 grams per day, to be supplemented by 1 kilogram of root crops and 125 grams of fresh fruit. In addition small amounts of sugar, tea, biscuits, and lard, and 500 grams of meat per week were to be supplied. The cost per labourer per year was calculated at 218 Mark. Not surprisingly, the New

165 Wendland 3.12.1908, RKA 2312: 30 ff
166 RKA 2311: 44-45. See also Firth, *New Guinea* 123-4 for a discussion of the ration debate.
167 Verordnung des Gouverneurs von Deutsch-Neuguinea, betr. die Ausführung und Anwerbung von Eingeborenen als Arbeiter in Deutsch Neuguinea, 4 March 1909 (with effect 1 January 1910). DKG 13: 147-53

Guinea Company protested loudly that proposed provisions were favouring labourers to the detriment of plantation owners, whose interests were ignored. Rations were seen as unrealistic, as it was impossible to provide the amounts of root crops and fresh fruit stipulated. They were neither available at local markets, nor was it possible to grow enough because of the shortage of labour and land.[168] The new labour ordinance was still under consideration when war broke out.

The New Guinea Company's objections were a singular demonstration of the failure of colonial plantation policies. After thirty years of colonisation, the labour force could not be supplied with nutritionally adequate rations. On recruitment labourers lost control over their food, and dietary improvements which would directly improve health and correspond closer to traditional foods were inimical to plantation interests. What land and labour there was had to be incorporated into the market economy, regardless of the effects on the health and welfare of the people.

The likelihood of the new ordinance being adopted remains conjectural. One key player, Governor Hahl, had left the colony in April 1914 and was replaced by Acting Governor Haber. If the new governor showed himself amenable to pressure from local plantation owners, this augured ill for the ordinance. Local companies were reacting strongly against the proposals, and there is no doubt of their powerful influence in the colony. However, another player had arrived in German New Guinea at the end of 1913, Dr Külz, the new Chief Medical Officer. His influence was never put to the test. His brief was public health in the colony, focusing on the health of the native population as the best guarantee for the development of the colonial economy. He would undoubtedly have fought for provisions to protect labourers as proposed in the draft ordinance.

Native Hospitals

By 1914 the health care system in German New Guinea included a number of native hospitals. The capital had a modern, well equipped native hospital which was opened on 1 April 1909, and in 1914 plans were well advanced to enlarge it.[169] In Kaewieng a hospital complex had been built in 1906.[170] In Namatanai the

---

168 Memorandum NGC to RKA 29 July 1914, RKA 2314: 8 ff
169 MB 1909/10: 505
170 A temporary native hospital built from bush material was taken into use in April 1904, and was replaced by a new hospital complex in 1906. MB 1911/12: 482-3. The dysentery barrack was due to be replaced in 1915.

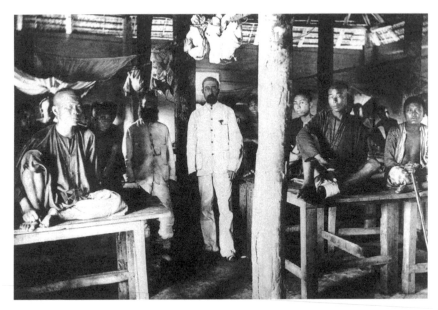

Native Hospital in Stephansort, late 1890s. Doctor, medical orderly and patients

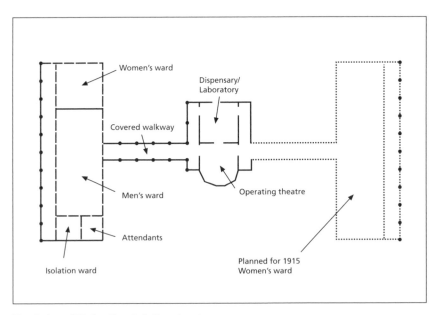

Sketchplan of Native Hospital, Namatanai

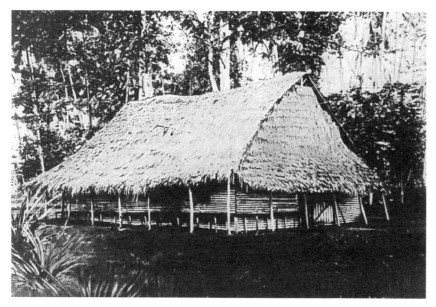

Temporary bush hospital in Namatanai

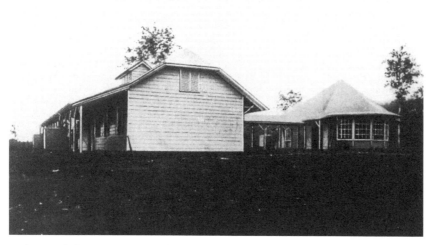

Native Hospital Namatanai, opened in 1912

first 40-bed stage of the native hospital was ready for occupation in January 1912, with the second stage of the hospital complex to be completed in 1915.[171] In Kieta, on Bougainville, the construction of a native hospital was begun in March 1914 to replace the temporary hospital built from bush material.[172] In Friedrich-Wilhelmshafen the New Guinea Company rebuilt the native hospital in 1903/04 on Beliao Island under the terms of agreement between the Reich and the company in connection with the transfer of the administration in 1899.[173] The building standard cannot have been high for the hospital quickly became the centre of dispute between the government and the company.[174] The latter was reluctant to carry out urgent repairs and build badly needed isolation wards. In a compromise solution the government built the isolation ward, and the company carried out some repairs so as to postpone replacement. In keeping with other centres in the colony, it was the government's responsibility to build and maintain a native hospital in Friedrich-Wilhelmshafen, but funds for a new complex became available only in 1913; the new hospital was completed when war broke out.[175]

Hospitals were the focus of the health care system and most of the doctors' work centred on them. Most of the day-to-day management was in the hands

---

171 A temporary building of bush material was set up to serve as hospital until the first wing of the hospital proper was ready in January 1912. This wing contained a large men's ward, a women's ward, a recovery room, and rooms for attendants. The windows of the women's ward were covered with iron bars. A covered walkway connected the wing with a smaller building containing the operating theatre, the dispensary and the laboratory. War intervened before plans for the second stage in 1915 came to fruition. A matching wing on the other side of the services building was to be the new women's ward. MB 1911/12: 481-2

172 Draft Annual Report 1913/14: 79

173 A tall, 37 metre long wooden barrack with corrugated iron roof and a cement floor, with a verandah around it and large windows, the building was subdivided into two sections: the larger one for men, some 28 m long, with 40 to 50 plank-beds, the smaller one for women with 15 to 20 beds. In the women's ward the windows were covered with fixed screens, and at night the doors were locked so as to "prevent contact between the two wards during the night". A covered cement path connected the main building with the operating/ treatment rooms and the dispensary. Outpatients were also treated in this building. The ancillary buildings consisted of ablutions, a house for the senior Chinese wardsmen, a kitchen with store and a room for the Melanesian 'boys', a small hut built from bush material for autopsies, a barrack with four or five beds, built entirely of corrugated iron to be used as an isolation ward, and several privies which were built directly over the water. One of the old barracks on Cutter Island was left standing as emergency accommodation in an epidemic. Several rain water tanks were installed as the water from the well near the hospital was suitable only for washing. AR 1907/08: 407-8

174 RKA 5770: 170

175 The new complex was similar to the old one—one large men's ward, a women's ward, operating theatre, dispensary, office, and outhouses. Draft AR 1913/14: 92

of a German medical orderly who supervised the work of the hospital attendants. He, in turn, was responsible to the doctor for his work. While this
organisation was in operation from the beginning, it was not formalised until
1911, when a formal duty statement for medical orderlies was issued in con-
junction with a duty statement for doctors.[176] In the early days the hospital
attendants were usually Chinese or Javanese, but after the turn of the century, local people were increasingly hired. There is little information on the
people who worked in hospitals, apart from names of medical orderlies (see
list Appendix IV). While in European hospitals women were charged with
the day-to-day management, native hospitals were the domain of men. The
majority of patients were men, but there is nothing to suggest who cared for
female patients, but it is possible that some attendants were women. As in
European hospitals, in the strictly hierarchical world of native hospitals, sub-
ordinates remained anonymous.

Hospitals absorbed a large share of the health care budget. They served to
isolate people with infectious diseases, and to care for the sick and injured.
With about 8 per cent of the labour force hospitalised at any one time in the
Bismarck Archipelago after the turn of the century, and higher during epidemics,[177] they fulfilled a useful function. Accustomed and trained to deal
with disease and injury in this manner, it is difficult to imagine that authorities would go about it in a different way in a colony. However, the main
health problems in the colony remained, with about the same malaria incidence after the turn of the century; epidemics of diarrhoeal diseases and
beriberi recurred in the labour force, and so did venereal infection. The question may be asked whether hospitals were favoured to the detriment of other
health care measures, and whether public works were neglected in favour of
hospitals. The government was faced with two different tasks: one was individual health care by providing facilities for nursing sick people; the other was
public health, the prevention of disease. Chronically short of funds, it had to
set priorities at all times—Berlin did not pour funds into the colony. In the
case of Rabaul the decision was to wait for a pleasant looking and well
equipped hospital, rather than waste funds on temporary sanitary facilities.
The situation was similar in all other centres. Confronted with the immediate need to care for large numbers of sick people, hospitals were built—cure
came before prevention.

176 *Amtsblatt* 1911: 183-4
177 MB 1906/07: 195. Before the turn of the century, the corresponding figure was around
    15%. *NKWL* 1898: 31-32; 37; AR 1898/99: 158

A labour force not immune to malaria, living on a poor diet, and in crowded and unsanitary conditions, created shocking conditions in Kaiser-Wilhelmsland. They were made worse by newcomers bringing in new diseases. Each year until the turn of the century, chances were that one out of six New Guinean plantation labourers working in Kaiser-Wilhelmsland would die. In the Bismarck Archipelago, where conditions were better, chances were about one in twenty-two,[178] and after the turn of the century, around one in thirty. If health conditions are judged by these figures, it is clear that gains were made and mortality rates similar to those in other Pacific plantation colonies started to become the norm.

In Kaiser-Wilhelmsland gains were pronounced, but the medical profession could take credit only for some of them. One was combatting smallpox: the epidemic, although brief, had had a considerable impact on labourers, but it was brought under control through vaccination and did not become endemic. Influenza epidemics in the early nineties had claimed uncounted numbers of labourers, but did not recur after these years. Much of the improvement in Kaiser-Wilhelmsland was therefore on account of these infections not recurring. Malaria was brought under limited control at the turn of the century, in Kaiser-Wilhelmsland and in the Bismarck Archipelago thus contributing to a better general state of health, so that people had more resistance to other diseases. The question is whether there was room for further improvement.

Regular recurrences of dysentery and beriberi suggest that standards of nutrition, water supply, and sanitary waste disposal were poor. While the government created a better environment for its labourers and police force in Rabaul with better housing, attention to water supply and sanitation, and dietary changes, similar improvements in other centres proceeded at a slow pace. Plantation owners, directly responsible for the conditions of a much larger labour force than the government, did little to imitate the hygienic standards set by the government in Rabaul. Until legislation, effective from 1 January 1910, came into force, there was no compulsion to do so, but even then there remains the question of how effectively the legislation could be policed. Like the government, the hard-headed plantation owners had grown used to relying on hospitals to take care of much of the ill health caused by poor conditions. But they could point to many fewer deaths compared with the early years, regardless of how these improvements had occurred. This no doubt

178 Based on figures by Shlomowitz, 'Pacific Labour Trade' 58

encouraged a notion that employers had done all that could be done for their labour force.

Hospitals were the focus of health care. Over the years the government built good native hospitals and expanded medical services. While there was unquestioning need for these services, there remains a nagging suspicion that they fostered the development of a hospital system at the expense of public health measures.

4

THE INDIGENOUS POPULATION

*If we don't succeed in increasing the native
population ... our economic progress in the colonies
will come to a halt. Therefore, native public health
is of foremost importance.*[1]

This chapter focuses on the indigenous population, the people who lived in villages and hamlets in districts under German control, to whom the Germans usually referred to as "free natives". The development of a public health policy, and strategies to integrate the indigenous population into government medical services form the topics of the first part of this chapter. The second part is a discussion of the question of population decline and growth.

The development of a public health policy proper began only after the Reich took over the administration of the colony in April 1899. Before that the New Guinea Company took measures as need arose, notably a ban on the sale of alcohol to natives, smallpox vaccination, and compulsory examination of labourers to prevent the spread of venereal infections.

The economic development of the colony, which depended on an increasing supply of labour, became the central concern of the Imperial administration. The refusal of Chinese and Dutch authorities to supply labour to the German colony, together with the unwillingness of planters to

---

1   L. Külz, 'Die seuchenhaften Krankheiten des Kindesalters der Eingeborenen und ihre Bedeutung für die koloniale Bevölkerungsfrage', *Koloniale Rundschau* 6(1913): 321-30

employ expensive Asian coolies[2] meant that the labour force had to come from within the colony. The population under German control—believed to be declining—was therefore seen as the colony's most valuable resource whose state of health became an important issue. As a declining population threatened the viability of the colony, population growth was essential for the future of the colony. Implicit in endeavours to create a healthy population was the role prescribed for New Guineans: men were to work for European masters, and women to bear and raise healthy children. Whether the native population had any rights within this grand scheme was a question which never arose.

HEALTH POLICIES AND STRATEGIES

Censuses

The basis for a native health policy was data on the size and health of the population. Census taking and health surveys became a continuing process; as a district came under government control, the population had to be counted and surveyed. Results of such surveys suggested two ways in which the administration could intervene: one was to change cultural practices; the other was to provide medical services to improve the health of the population, an improvement which in turn would contribute to population growth. A third option, strict limitations on recruitment, was politically not feasible.

The two aspects of this approach were interdependent and concurrent and closely connected with numerical and health surveys. Without population data, no long term economic plans could be made. Without a general health assessment it was not possible to determine what needed to be done to curb the population decline and improve health. However, without cultural change, practices inhibiting population increase could not be eradicated, nor was it possible to introduce western medical services and public health measures, such as personal hygiene or the use of unpolluted water. Yet, without improvements in public health and medical intervention, the population

---

2   Firth, *New Guinea* 116-18. Governor Hahl advocated Asian immigration throughout his tenure, and envisaged "a melting pot of Asiatic and Melanesian races". See John Moses, 'Imperial German Priorities in New Guinea 1885-1914' in S. Latukefu, ed., *Papua New Guinea: a century of colonial impact, 1884-1984*, (Port Moresby: NRI, 1989) 163-178

could not grow. One more aspect became increasingly obvious: without considerable financial investment, effective intervention was not possible.

Doctors were closely involved in this work. Not only did they accompany district officers to count heads and survey health; doctors had to attend to health problems and, most importantly, individual treatment had to be successful so as to convince others to make use of the services offered. The 'selling' of western ideas on health and medicine proved a most difficult aspect of doctors' work. Missions, interested in population growth for reasons of their own, cooperated closely with the administration and doctors on many aspects of what was seen as "the population problem", and were also influential in shaping perceptions of this problem.

The first population census was taken in 1898 on the Neulauenburg islands (Duke of York group), the first people in the Bismarck Archipelago to come under the influence of a mission, the Methodist Mission, which had set up there in 1875. The mission had kept records of its flock for years, and missionaries were very much involved in the census; they knew the people and therefore reasonably accurate figures could be obtained. Population counts were again made there in 1900, 1903, 1907 and 1911, with the last two considered to be reasonably reliable, as distinctions between adults and children were made with the help of mission records.[3]

By 1914 the population had been counted or estimated in most of the areas under German control. Doctors from naval ships and missionaries often assisted. Dr Besenbruch's[4] experience was probably typical of the procedure. While the survey ship *Planet* was on an oceanographic survey of the north coast of New Britain, he was charged with surveying the villages on Lolobau island and from there west along the coast to the Willaumez Peninsula. This district had had little direct contact with Europeans with the exception of limited recruitment. In villages where some men had worked on plantations, the doctor found it reasonably easy to get people together; ex-labourers cooperated, interpreting and encouraging villagers to gather. Counting heads and taking a look was about all that Besenbruch was usually able to do. In villages where no one had worked for Europeans and even the interpreter could not understand the language, the doctor glimpsed women and children disappear into the bush, and only a few men remained to be listed. In some villages everybody disappeared and did not show up even if Besenbruch waited for hours. The census categories were simply men and women, boys and girls

3   Von Seckendorff report, 23.10.1903. RKA 7434:42; 63-64
4   A naval doctor on the survey ship *Planet*. Report in *Amtsblatt* 1912: 195; 200-9; 243-48

(age based on a visual judgement), and health assessments were superficial. Nevertheless, Besenbruch noted some clear differences: some villages and hamlets had good plantations and the population looked quite vigorous; others had a general look of neglect and people appeared to be in poor health. In such places the large number of adults with smallpox scars were conspicuous; some were blind in one or both eyes, probably because of smallpox which had spread to the Nakanai region fifteen years earlier.[5] Yaws was prevalent in children, skin diseases affected most people; some had ulcers, a few filariasis, two were leprosy suspects. He heard or saw nothing of dysentery, but suspected that two or three people were infected with tuberculosis.

The general state of health among the Nakanai people was typical of many populations on New Britain, as a survey by Kopp confirmed some months later.[6] In this doctor's opinion there were no problems that could not be overcome with medical services and a good water supply. The Nakanai people undoubtedly represented a useful population pool, a resource to be maintained and integrated into the plantation economy.

After the first census, head taxes were imposed and population recount and tax collection were combined. The doctor accompanied the district officer on his rounds and, while census and tax lists were checked, heads counted and money collected, the doctor carried out medical examinations. Accuracy of the first count varied a great deal; in areas which had little contact with Europeans, the first census was known to be not much more than a rough estimate.

Just how erroneous a first census could be was well demonstrated on the Vitu islands. The 1911 census showed a population of 527 on Unea, the southern-most island of the group. A recount in 1913 showed a total of 1070 people, 391 men, 357 women, 213 boys and 109 girls. As there were strong suspicions that children had been hidden during that poll, the population was recounted six months later, and a total of 1399 people were found to be living on the island—490 men, 439 women, 293 boys and 177 girls. At this latest count the district officer was satisfied that at long last all heads of this "refractory" people had been counted, and that the overall population of the Vitu islands was 2523 people—867 men, 794 women, 516 boys, 346 girls.[7]

---

5   M. Rascher, 'Auf der Suche nach Pocken', *Hiltruper Monatshefte* 1898: 229-34
6   K. Kopp, 'Zur Frage des Bevölkerungsrückgangs in Neupommern', *ASTH* 17(1913): 729-50
7   *Amtsblatt* 1913: 272; 1914: 47

Malaria

With malaria as the main health problem, attempts were made to come to grips with the problem in the native population after the turn of the century. The results that Professor Koch obtained late in 1899 at Bogadjim station from blood testing and quinine therapy among labourers encouraged him in the belief that malaria could be eradicated in villages through systematic quinine therapy, a belief reinforced by results obtained in Wilhelmshaven in northwest Germany.[8] To confirm this theory, Dr Dempwolff, who had worked in New Guinea from 1895-97, was sent back for further field work and to repeat Koch's experiments and attempt malaria eradication in the indigenous population. Dempwolff found that the promising results obtained by Koch with quinine therapy had been completely negated by renewed severe attacks of malaria, and Bogadjim had reverted to the same malaria centre it had been before Koch's arrival.[9]

Further work in Kaiser-Wilhelmsland and the Gazelle Peninsula convinced Dempwolff that quinine therapy was not a practicable way to eradicate malaria. Unless enormous sums of money were made available, sums which would bear no relationship to the economic value of the region, it was a hopeless undertaking.[10] The topography of the country with its widely dispersed villages and hamlets created great logistic difficulties. Without proper transport—no suitable horse was available for Dempwolff—it was an arduous enterprise to get to the dispersed villages and there to screen people for malaria parasites and to supervise a regular quinine intake. Blood testing for malaria parasites was slow and time-consuming; as he was hampered by eye problems, Dempwolff was able to analyse only about twenty to twenty-five slides a day. Dr Wendland, who was working with him was recalled to Herbertshöhe after a few weeks.[11] Although Dempwolff thought that it was theoretically possible to eradicate malaria with quinine therapy and prophylaxis, he realised that the practical problems were beyond the capabilities of one man. He therefore decided to concentrate on establishing the incidence of malaria and tracing its spread over the last few years.

Focusing on the Gazelle Peninsula and islands in the Bismarck Archipelago,

---

8   R. Koch, 'Die Bekämpfung der Malaria', *Zeitschrift für Hygiene und Infektionskrankheiten* 43(1902): 4

9   O. Dempwolff, 'Malaria-Expedition' 47(1904): 89. See W.H. Ewers, 'Malaria in the early years of German New Guinea', for a detailed analysis and tables of Dempwolff's findings.

10   Dempwolff, 'Malaria-Expedition', 123

11   Dempwolff's private letter to Koch, 23.9.1902. Robert-Koch-Institut

Dempwolff found that infestation varied a great deal, from heavy on Cape Birara (Cape Gazelle) to sporadic in the Simpsonhafen district and even malaria-free districts. In at least two districts that were free on first testing in October 1902, he was able to observe the "local advance" of malaria. One was Gunamba,[12] where a Catholic mission station was set up in 1898. When retesting three hamlets there he found that five of eight children under the age of five, and five of twenty ranging between six and ten years had parasites in their blood. As a group of labourers had returned from Kaiser-Wilhelmsland very recently, it was assumed that they had brought the infection back to the villages. When Father Eberlein from the Sacred Heart Mission set up the station, he noticed that people in this district rarely had malaria, and that it was not unusual to meet a woman with five or six children, whereas along the coast women seemed to have at most two.[13] He could not, of course, understand the implications of his observation, as the connection between malaria and infant mortality was not then known.

In the previously malaria-free Gunanur district, where a Wesleyan Mission station was established, Dempwolff also found malaria in March 1903, where there had been none six months earlier. This recent infection was ascribed to increased traffic between villages because of pacification.[14] The Crater Peninsula was also found to be malaria-free in 1903. Five years later Dr Wick found severe malaria infestation with parasites and enlarged spleens in children and adults.[15] Whether infection in all these districts was by returning labourers who had acquired it in a malarial region, increasing traffic among villages, or missionaries cannot be established. What is certain is that colonisation had ramifications visibly detrimental to health.

The speed with which malaria affected a population was clearly demonstrated in the population of the Western Islands (Ninigo Group). On Ninigo, Dempwolff observed that, among others, the high chief was infected with malaria and very sick. The high mortality (between thirty and forty people in the six months before his visit to the atoll), led him to conclude that malaria had been introduced only very recently and that it, not venereal disease as was casually assumed, was the health problem that plagued the islanders. To the east in the Hermit Group Dempwolff found only two people with enlarged

---

12 A high plateau, about 5 kilometres inland from the coast, half way between Malapaua and Vunakokor on the Gazelle Peninsula

13 *DKB* 10(1899): 628

14 Dempwolff, 'Malaria-Expedition', 97

15 Wick report 18.1.1909, RKA 2311: 130

spleens and one man infested with malaria parasites. As it turned out, this man had been in Herbertshöhe recently as a witness in a court case, and the doctor suggested that he had become infected there. As the atoll was infested with anopheles, Dempwolff thought it highly likely that the non-immune population would be devastated by malaria.

When Dempwolff examined the population on Wuvulu (west of the Ninigo Group) late in 1903 he found that 90 per cent of people of all ages had grossly enlarged spleens and around 40 per cent of those examined were malaria infected. The whole population looked sickly, there were few small children, and during his two week stay on the island at the end of 1902, he never saw a baby or a pregnant woman. He was sure that malaria had been introduced in 1899 when a trader together with a number of labourers from Eitape settled on the anopheles infested atoll. The population, in the past estimated at around 2000 to 2500, was reduced to under 1000, many having died in the first eight months of the year. An examination of two women said to suffer from the same symptoms as those who had died, showed bronchopneumonia. Dempwolff speculated that people weakened by malaria were highly susceptible to respiratory tract infections. The Wuvuluans, at a time when they were severely weakened by malaria and vulnerable to other diseases, had been encouraged by the trader Leonhard to spend long periods fishing for the increasingly valuable trochus shells, and long exposure predisposed them to respiratory tract infections. Another factor likely to contribute to the death toll was the poor huts in two of the villages. Two years earlier the island's high chief Puala had had these villages destroyed when the people refused to pay their tribute so that, instead of their traditional, carefully constructed houses, they lived in poorly built huts that offered little protection from the weather. Poor living conditions increased their susceptibility to pneumonia. Dempwolff expected further deaths on the island, as a tidal wave at the end of November, just before his arrival, had destroyed two villages, and exposed malaria-weakened villagers to the weather.[16]

The population on Wuvulu had been struck by three misfortunes in four years: malaria, internal strife, and natural disaster. The first was directly due to advancing colonial interests, and was undoubtedly the most devastating. Internal strife and natural disasters were probably not unusual, and even if they did check the population, they did not have long-term effects. The introduction of malaria was different: it destroyed the islanders health, and those who survived were

16 Dempwolff, 'Ueber aussterbende Völker: die Eingeborenen der "westlichen Inseln" in Deutsch-Neu-Guinea', *Zeitschrift für Ethnologie* 36(1904): 395-413

weakened and less resistant to other stress. The consequence was an enormous population loss, so large that Dempwolff doubted that the Wuvuluans could recover unless, as a first priority, malaria was eradicated. But, as he asked wistfully, who was going to foot an annual bill of around 30,000 Mark for a malaria eradication program for a thousand savages?[17] As Firth commented, there were planters ready to benefit and take what the dead left behind.[18]

This is not to imply that the government fostered deliberate extermination. While it was technically possible to eradicate malaria on this island because of its isolation, there were two obstacles. One, as Dempwolff realised, was financial; the second was the presence of German plantation and trading interests, a point on which Dempwolff remained silent. But, if anything, these were obstacles even harder to overcome than malaria.[19]

Dempwolff found improvement in the health situation in only one region since Koch had been there three years earlier. This was the Kaewieng district where, instructed by Koch, district officer Boluminski and his wife dispensed quinine to natives in surrounding villages. While the distribution was not systematic, Dempwolff found that it helped to reduce the incidence of infection appreciably.[20] However, when Dr Hoffmann carried out extensive examinations in 1907, about one third of the men and boys examined in villages around Kaewieng had enlarged spleens and suffered severe malaria attacks, a discovery which was puzzling. Was malaria constantly reintroduced or was it seasonal? Hoffmann was unable to decide but hoped that, as many people were already familiar with the benefits of quinine, others could also be persuaded to take it.[21]

---

17 Dempwolff, "Ueber aussterbende Völker' 413
18 Firth, *New Guinea* 115
19 The possibility of population extermination by planters was raised by the Colonial Office in 1908 in connection with an agreement between Forsayth & Company and the government in Rabaul. The clause that gave rise to concern in Berlin stipulated that should natives die out within 30 years, the government was obliged to hand over the native reserves to the owners of the island free of charge. The Colonial Office pointed out that such a condition could lead an unscrupulous owner to work towards the extinction of a people. As the population on Nukumanu atoll (Tasman Island) had declined from around 300 people in 1900 to 94 in 1909, there was justification for concern. Following his inspection tour, district officer Dr Klug opined that there was no cause for alarm as the Forsayth man was of good character; furthermore, it was not in the interest of the company to exterminate the remaining population, as they were a valuable labour force which prepared copra cheaply for the company. Nevertheless, in order to ensure that the situation remained satisfactory, Klug suggested that the district officer should pay an annual visit to the island. RKA 2431: 91 ff
20 Dempwolff, 'Malaria-Expedition' 124
21 Hoffmann report to Governor, 21.10.1907. RKA 2310: 90 f.

The realisation that malaria was spreading inexorably, and that eradication was impossible, convinced Dempwolff that the focus had to be shifted. Instead of trying to eradicate malaria in the whole population, emphasis had to be placed on protecting colonists by creating malaria-free zones. To a gathering of settlers he explained that systematic quinine therapy for all infected people living or working in or near European households would eradicate malaria in the immediate surroundings of such households. In order to keep these surroundings malaria-free, quinine had to be dispensed regularly as a prophylactic measure. The malaria battle was a continuing one and had to be taken up by individual households and institutions.[22] As discussed in the previous chapter, this proposal met with passive resistance or indifference from Europeans. In the end Dempwolff concluded that systematic quininisation failed because of the difficult access to the indigenous population—both geographically and because of their low level of civilisation—the indolence of Europeans, too large a fluctuation among labourers, and the vast areas that were malaria infested.[23] In other words, malaria eradication was a difficult and complex set of problems and a quick bacteriological solution, as Koch had envisaged, was not possible. At this point the concept of malaria-free zones was taken one step further: races had to live apart so that infected and untreatable blacks would not infect whites. Racial segregation was applied to a certain extent when Kaewieng was built, and became central to the planning of the new capital Rabaul,[24] as related earlier. To protect white families on individual settlements, natives' dwellings and labourers' quarters were shifted well away from the owner's residence to ensure a cordon sanitaire.[25]

Dysentery

On the Gazelle Peninsula dysentery was seen as the major affliction for natives. Laboratory tests established that most epidemics were bacillary, but the 1909 outbreak was amoebic.[26] Old settlers remembered that the first dysentery outbreak among natives followed the return of the recruiting ship *Lord of the Islands*

---

22 'The malaria situation on the Gazelle Peninsula', a talk given on 29 May 1903 in Herbertshöhe. Archives Robert-Koch-Institut

23 Dempwolff, 'Malaria-Expedition' 126

24 Koch had foreshadowed racial segregation in his talk before the British Medical Congress in 1901, when listing the four ways in which malaria in Europeans could be prevented. T.D. Brock, *Robert Koch: A Life in Medicine and Bacteriology* (Madison: Science Tech Publications, 1986) 250

25 MB 1908/09: 367

26 Wick, *Amtsblatt* 1909: 51

from Queensland in the early 1880s, from which labourers disembarked south of Blanche Bay on the St. George Channel.[27] Dysentery remained endemic and German doctors stationed at Herbertshöhe from 1896 regularly reported epidemics, the "scourge of the native population". A devastating epidemic affected the north coast of the Gazelle Peninsula, and some areas of New Ireland in 1899. The Quarantine Legislation, amended in that year to include dysentery as a quarantinable disease,[28] did nothing to reduce its incidence. It was not until 1908 that the administration began to take some effective measures with the installation of wells in some villages. Following a particularly severe epidemic in the previous year when dysentery crossed the whole of the Gazelle Peninsula from east to west in a six months period, Dr Wendland proposed that the government could improve hygienic conditions for natives "without too much cost" through the installation of artesian wells in the larger villages.[29] He was not sanguine about the likely improvements in the health situation because of the "low cultural level" of the population, and suggested that missions should cooperate and teach their flock basic personal hygiene. Wendland's reservations suggest that the delay in building wells was connected with doctors' expectations of what villagers would be able to learn and adopt, but their differing views of the effect of polluted water on health also played a part. Wendland and Danneil debated this question for five years and finally agreed that the quality of the drinking water was crucial and therefore, as a first step, water supplies had to be improved. However, as infection by flies, contaminated food and direct person to person cross-infection were other ways of spreading the disease, the threat of recurring dysentery epidemics remained.

Even then, progress on well construction was slow as "funds [did] not permit large-scale measures".[30] By 1911 eight wells had been dug in Rabaul (in the Melanesian, Malay and Chinese quarters, and at the native hospital) and ten in villages on the Gazelle Peninsula. On Matupi there were technical problems; drilling tests everywhere produced salty or sulphurous ground water. In other districts, little seems to have been done in this respect, apart from sinking wells on stations, with the exception of Manus where seven wells were built in 1912. The speed with which a bacillary dysentery epidemic spread throughout the villages early in 1912 and killed one in seven

---

27   *NKWL* 1897: 39, Wendland. There was some debate whether dysentery was endemic before the arrival of Europeans; Koch considered it an introduced disease. AR 1899/1900: 186.

28   Ergänzung zur Quarantäne Verordnung vom 29. September 1891. 19 August, 1899, *DKG* 4: 93-4

29   MB 1907/08: 417

30   AR 1908/09: 297

people in fifteen coastal villages, required more than crisis management. The first step was a clean water supply which meant that open water holes in the villages had to be filled in and proper wells had to be constructed.[31] In the Rabaul district the administration also tried to persuade villagers to change burial customs and to adopt "hygienically sound" burials.[32]

Dysentery outbreaks were not restricted to the relatively densely populated Gazelle Peninsula. On his trip to Buka and Bougainville in 1914, Leber found that dysentery was endemic on these islands. He contended that this was "undoubtedly the source of contagion" from which infection was regularly carried by new recruits to the Gazelle Peninsula, and that the outbreak on Manus in 1912 could clearly be traced back to the newly arrived labourers from Buka.[33] All the evidence strongly suggests that dysentery was going to remain a protracted problem.

Medical Services for Villagers

The integration of the population into the medical service was seen as essential if population growth was to be achieved, but this presented certain difficulties. The centralised medical system such as the Germans had established by building hospitals in European centres did not lend itself to serve the widely dispersed population. For a doctor to travel to remote areas to undertake routine treatment of minor complaints—best carried out at village level— was time-consuming. In any case, there was usually enough work at the hospitals to keep doctors occupied. More importantly, because of the distances involved, doctors were unable to intervene rapidly in frequent outbreaks of dysentery. It was therefore essential that another way be found to get into villages and bring in health services. Such a village-based system, it was realised, demanded a large number of medical and para-medical staff to live among village people for extended periods.

The second, even more fundamental question was how to impose European medicine, familiarise the population with it and get villagers to make more use of the services provided. Neither the best equipped hospital nor the best doctor were of any use if people could not be persuaded to avail themselves of the service offered. Superstitions and ignorance were seen as serious impediments to the adoption of western medicine. The term superstition (*Aberglaube*)

---

31 Kopp, 'Bericht über die Dysenterie-Bekämpfung in Manus', *Amtsblatt* 1912: 151-4
32 AR 1912/13: 360
33 A. Leber, 'Centrale Durchquerung der Insel Manus' (May 1914), unpublished manuscript: 6

encompassed many differing beliefs about causes of illness and death that doctors came across. By continuously demonstrating the efficacy and superiority of their techniques, doctors hoped to foment changes in attitudes. What they attempted was no less than a cultural revolution by imposing a fundamental change in the values and attitudes of New Guineans. Meanwhile, doctors' frustrations were summed up by Dr Danneil when he lamented that:

> Villagers make up only a small percentage of our patients. A Melanesian consults a doctor willingly only in exceptional circumstances. His indifference towards his own body and his utter lack of understanding of the causes of illness, his disinclination to leave his family for any length of time, his reluctance to give up his dirty kanaka habits and to submit to certain systematic rules and modes of behaviour, together with his very limited horizon prevent him from making use of free medical treatment.[34]

This outburst showed the points at which cultures clashed. Doctors assumed that natives should and would readily accept the benefits of colonisation. But, instead of putting their trust in doctors, accepting their intervention and western scientific and technological achievements, natives clung to their old ways. In every district the situation was similar: villagers were suspicious and shy; then a few could be persuaded to see a doctor, usually because of ulcers or a severe injury, even for quinine against a severe fever attack, but not for other internal conditions. Villagers knew about doctors and hospitals because compulsory medical examination of all recruits meant that all who signed up as labourers were forced to come into contact with European doctors. If labourers fell sick during their indenture—and most did—they were hospitalised and medical treatment was unavoidable. An increasing number of people came into contact with European medicine in this way. This may in part explain why some sought medical aid in cases where treatment was obviously beneficial. They had observed and experienced that many traumas, ulcers, skin infections and venereal disease could be healed. But they had also seen people die in hospitals—those who had survived the early 1890s in Kaiser-Wilhelmsland carried horrendous memories of death and disease. They had seen enough deaths in hospitals to know that doctors were not all-powerful, knowledge they were bound to share with their fellow-villagers. It should therefore not have been a surprise that indigenous people were reluctant to seek medical treatment, and that they chose the circumstances under which they would consult a doctor.

Experience showed that villagers near stations made little—and selective—

34 MB 1904/05: 198

use of hospitals. In Herbertshöhe, where missions were able to influence people and encouraged them to make use of doctors and hospitals, only sixteen people were hospitalised in 1905/6.[35] By 1910/11 the number hospitalised had risen to sixty, some with complicated fractures or serious injuries.[36] More came to the hospital as outpatients: about one hundred in 1903/4;[37] with the number steadily increasing to 365 in 1910/11, a number seen as signalling that medical activity was gaining the trust of the local population.[38] That the demand by outpatients was growing, but selective, is exemplified in an analysis of the patients treated from 1 July to 30 September 1913 at Herbertshöhe native hospital: a total of 209 came to the clinic, 65 men, 59 women, and 85 children. They were treated for the following complaints: 180 ulcers, 9 scabies, 4 middle ear infection, 3 bronchitis, 3 burns, 3 rheumatism, 2 yaws, 2 conjunctivitis, 1 venereal granuloma, 1 tissue inflammation, and 1 fractured arm.[39] Nearly nine out of ten cases came for ulcers. This proportion was not always quite so high, as figures for the first quarter of 1914 suggest: of the 339 outpatients about six out of ten were treated for ulcers. The other cases were: 38 skin complaints (scabies, ringworm), 38 eye infections, 34 rheumatism, 10 bronchitis, 5 malaria, 3 venereal granuloma, 2 inflammation of neck glands, 2 burns, 1 each ear infection, tissue inflammation, abrasion, inflammation of testes, inflammation of knee joint, and growth on hand.[40] A doctor had been in Herbertshöhe for eighteen years since Dr Danneil started work there in January 1896—creating a demand for the medical service had been a long slow process, and even after this time a doctor was not in very great demand.

As often as work at native hospitals permitted, doctors made the rounds of villages. On Matupi urgent intervention was needed when trachoma flared up in mid-1908. Doctors had not enough time to carry out the regular and lengthy treatment, and the help of Father Bögershausen from the Sacred Heart Mission was invoked. Although the epidemic was brought under control, a few cases were found again in 1911.[41] The sudden appearance of trachoma

35 MB 1905/06: 255

36 MB 1910/11: 624

37 MB 1903/04: 180. The figures are for the number of patients, not the number of cases; each patient may well have paid several visits to the clinic.

38 MB 1910/11: 625

39 Runge report, RKA 5772: 280-1

40 Runge report, RKA 5773: 89-90

41 Born report RKA 5771: 45; Wick RKA 3774: 35. Drs. Prowacek and Leber spent a few days in the Rabaul district on their way to Saipan and Samoa to carry out research into the many eye diseases there and confirmed the diagnosis by Born and Wick. Report by Leber and Prowacek 1.6.1911, RKA 6045. Also G. Bögershausen, 'Die Augenkrankheit auf der Gazelle-Halbinsel', *Hiltruper Monatshefte* 4(1912): 356. For the work of Leber and Prowacek in Saipan and Samoa see G. Kluxen, *Augenheilkunde deutscher Tropenärzte vor 1918* (Düsseldorf: Triltsch, 1980)

raised serious concerns and doctors were instructed to pay careful attention to eye infections as neglect could lead to blindness. As it was suspected that trachoma had been introduced by Chinese, instructions were issued that their medical examination on arrival had to include an eye examination.[42]

Doctors were not surprised that pneumonia and pleurisy were frequent, in particular at the onset of the rainy season and following a big *singsing*, and claimed many victims. Natives danced and sang all night, then, exhausted and covered in sweat, slept in the open. "No wonder", one doctor commented, "there are so many pulmonary infections".[43]

The government was well aware of the medical work done by missions and missionaries and doctors co-operated in persuading villagers to use medical services; missionaries sent seriously ill patients to the hospital, or called the doctor in an emergency. From 1908 onwards, on the initiative of Dr Born, missions were supplied with bandages and medications free of cost for the use in the care of natives. This was done with the clear understanding that patients would be told that supplies were from the government and free of charge. The government was not going to lose an opportunity to demonstrate its generosity towards the native population. The question of charging for medical treatment came up repeatedly. Generally speaking, doctors were in favour of a free medical service in the belief that it would encourage people to use it when necessary. The government was inclined to make small charges, especially from people living in the Herbertshöhe area who could well afford it. Overall, no clear policy was ever developed and costs were absorbed within the hospital budget.[44]

Missionaries were especially helpful in reporting suspected cases of leprosy. The first case was a man from the Astrolabe Plains. Apart from confirming the diagnosis with laboratory tests, and some treatment which improved the man's general condition, there was not much that could be done for him, and he was sent back to his village. The villagers were informed of the nature of the illness and instructed to isolate the man or have as little contact with him as possible. Another two cases, one a woman from Bogia (Potsdamhafen district), the other from Ruo, were found around the same time.[45] Two years later two cases were reported from the hinterland of Friedrich-Wilhelmshafen. A man from Lambom Island (off Cape St. George, southern New Ireland), a boy in the Kaewieng district, and a man in the Herbertshöhe

---

42 Circular from Hahl to all doctors, 8 July 1908, together with instructions by Born on how to recognise and treat trachoma. RKA 5952: 77-78

43 MB 1909/10: 504

44 Wick, RKA 5771: 128

45 MB 1908/09: 399-400

district, were also found with leprosy around that time.[46] The few reported cases suggest that leprosy was rare, but there were enough to provoke the governor to issue instructions to all doctors that during visits to villages particular attention was to be paid to leprosy; cases should be isolated in specially built huts near native hospitals, and treatment with Nastin or Antileprol was to be carried out in all cases confirmed by laboratory tests.[47] Not all doctors agreed that isolation was appropriate or humane;[48] nor was it practicable: the leper patient isolated in Herbertshöhe absconded several times and returned to his village. Two newly discovered leprosy cases, a young man from Paparatawa and a boy in Kaewieng, were therefore put in the care of missions in the hope that the missionaries might be able to exert better control.[49] No decision on how to deal with leprosy patients was ever made, but it became obvious that missions would have to be involved if the government insisted on quarantining them.

To overcome shortages in staff and the distrust of the native population, Dr Born, who worked in Herbertshöhe and Rabaul from May 1908 to the end of 1909, proposed a scheme similar to the one he had developed on Yap (in the Carolines).[50] The basis of the scheme was to involve indigenous people in the delivery of some basic health services in villages. Men were to undergo training in the native hospitals for around three months; thereafter they would be equipped with bandages and medications, and set up for medical work in their villages. The proposal had obvious merits: a native medical assistant—eventually known as *Heiltultul* [medical *tultul*]—would accustom people to European methods of dealing with illness, to the use of medications and bandages. He would act as a "pioneer" who familiarised people with new ideas about disease, and inculcate trust in western medical practices and doctors,[51] preparing villagers for doctors to carry out more complex tasks. The medical *tultul* would also report epidemics or severe illness that needed more specific help. The cost of the scheme would be small.

Training of young men began almost immediately in the Rabaul native hospital. They were taught basic treatment of wounds, ulcers, and the com-

---

46   MB 1909/10: 494; MB 1910/11: 643

47   *Gesundheitswesen*: 78-79

48   MB 1908/09: 399-400

49   MB 1909/10: 494; MB 1910/11: 643

50   Born report for period 11.5.-30.6.1908, RKA 5771: 45. For Born's work on Yap see W.U. Eckart, 'Medicine and German colonial expansion in the Pacific', in R. MacLeod, ed. *Disease, Medicine and Empire: Perspectives on western medicine and the experience of European expansion*, (London: Routledge, 1988) 86-7

51   MB 1911/12: 494

mon ringworm, and the rudiments of dispensing quinine and other medications for respiratory tract and gastro-enteric diseases. After training, the *Heiltultul* was ready to set up his post in a small bush hut, equipped with a medical chest containing bandages and a few medications such as Dermatol, Styrax, both used for the treatment of skin diseases, liquid quinine, castor oil, an expectorant, carbolic soap and other antiseptics and disinfectants. One year later three villages had a medical *tultul*—Matupi, Tavui and Raluana, all in the vicinity of Rabaul. Within the next twelve months three were settled in the Duke of York group, eight in the Rabaul district, and another three were in training. In the Kaewieng district there were twenty medical *tultul* by 1912.[52]

Doctors found quickly that a *tultul* could not carry out effective work unless he had "a certain standing" in his village.[53] This suggests that the system could not function without cooperation at village level. It was not enough for a *tultul* to know how to treat ulcers or dispense medications; without the sanction of other villagers he could not apply his skills; his standing was not gained from training as a *tultul*; he had to be well regarded in his village before training. Experience showed also that training needed to be longer than three months, preferably one year, with a short stint at a native hospital for further training about a year later. Regular inspection tours by the doctor or the medical orderly ensured that *tultuls* were competently carrying out their work.[54] By 1914 there were over 130 *tultuls*.[55] By that time the plan was to train forty men annually, so that a complete network could be established throughout the pacified areas.[56]

The scheme did not operate long enough to be fully developed, and because of the short period of its operation, it is difficult to assess its impact. From scant information it is clear that doctors were satisfied with the way in which the scheme was shaping. In Kaewieng Dr Hoffmann[57] found that the *tultuls* did useful work in dispensing quinine and in managing outbreaks

52   MB 1909/10: 503-4; 1911/12: 494
53   MB 1912/13: 51
54   The experience on Manus in 1913—where 10 *tultul* were installed after 3 months training at Rabaul—confirmed that this training period was insufficient and longer training together with retraining was necessary. (Draft AR 1913/14: 65) The situation was similar in the south of New Ireland; following an inspection some of the *tultul* were taken back to the Namatanai hospital for further training. Braunert report, 16.1.1914, RKA 5773: 22
55   At least 18 in the Rabaul district (which included the Duke of York Group); at least 20 in Kaewieng, 85 in Namatanai, 10 on Manus
56   Draft Budget 1915. G255/754
57   MB 1911/12: 497

of dysentery. In order to deal with such outbreaks they were taught to isolate patients in a special hut, to observe basic hygiene with the safe disposal of faeces, and to treat patients with castor oil and Antidysentericum and plenty of sweet tea. They were also instructed on the importance of clean water. Hoffmann was also gratified when one of the *tultul* sent women suffering from gonorrhoea to him for treatment. The referral of patients for treatment of more serious complaints, especially venereal disease, was a much hoped for response.

On Manus the dysentery epidemic in 1912 gave the impetus to train *tultuls*.[58] With only one medical orderly on the island, a support system was essential if any medicine was to reach villagers. More than anything, the authorities feared another dysentery outbreak; and *tultuls* were the first line of defence.

The system was most developed in Namatanai, with eighty-five *tultuls* working there in 1914.[59] Some time after the station had been set up in 1904, station manager Wostrack, by training a medical orderly, began to teach some native men to apply dressings and other minor treatments. Necessity may have forced him to train native assistants, as no other assistant was on the station for any length of time. Training ceased, apparently because of the increased work load on the station manager.[60] There is little information on Wostrack's work, but the people trained by him may have been the core group to work in villages when Dr Kröning took up duties in Namatanai in 1911.

The scheme seemed to work in that villagers became accustomed to European medications in a limited way and with it learned a different way of dealing with some diseases. The *tultul* was the champion of Western medicine but his activities were circumscribed by his personal standing in his community. Nevertheless, doctors were apparently happy with the way the project was evolving and there are indications that it came to be seen as more than just the means of paving the way for doctors: in time it would be the basis for the development of a system of well-trained indigenous paramedical staff who would not only treat ulcers and hand out cough medicine, quinine and Antidysentericum, but would also be involved in the all important education in hygiene at village level.

Heiltultuls were certainly cheap. The government paid a *tultul* 20 Mark per year, and the cost of restocking his medicine chest was estimated to be about

58   Kopp, 'Dysenterie-Bekämpfung,' 153
59   Braunert report 16.1.1914, RKA 5773: 21
60   MB 1911/12: 495

75 Mark per year, a total annual cost of roughly 100 Mark per *tultul*. Curiously, a medical *tultul* was paid the same wage during his traineeship at the hospital, where he had free board and lodging, as he received when he was working in a village.[61] This suggests that he was not expected to work full time in his medical capacity. Yet it appears that there was enough work to keep him occupied, which created a ludicrous situation, as a man could earn three times as much in a year working on a plantation.[62] However, there is some indication that *tultuls* were exempt from compulsory public works and from recruitment,[63] which may have acted as an incentive to train as a *tultul*.

In Friedrich-Wilhelmshafen the situation differed from that in the Bismarck Archipelago. People resorted even less to a doctor. Although the people in Kaiser-Wilhelmsland had no objection to smallpox vaccination, they resisted medical aid except for ulcer treatment. Even then, patients were likely to stop coming for treatment when they thought they were cured, rather than waiting for the doctor to judge treatment as complete.[64] Hospitalisation was virtually impossible, as people refused to share a room with people from other districts. Young men who had worked for Europeans were expected to be more amenable to western ideas, yet they still remained under the influence of village elders and thus captives to village beliefs.[65] Dr Liesegang, an ex-military doctor who started work in Friedrich-Wilhelmshafen in April 1910, frustrated at the lack of response by villagers to his visits, decided upon forceful intervention. Accompanied by police troops, and equipped with a list made out by the district officer, the doctor went from village to village and called people up for medical inspection. Those seen to require medical treatment, usually for ulcers and yaws, were treated on the spot or, depending on the severity of the condition, taken to Friedrich-Wilhelmshafen, where huts were provided to accommodate them as outpatients. The results of these outings were poor, for in the first year he brought a total of only forty-four people to Friedrich-Wilhelmshafen in this way, and thirty-one in the following twelve months. Realising that this method did not achieve its desired ends, and strongly suspecting that seriously ill people were kept hidden, Liesegang suggested that a second doctor should be based in Madang, to work as a travelling doctor; his sporadic short visits achieved little.[66] There is nothing to suggest that training of medical *tultuls* was taken up in Friedrich-Wilhelmshafen. In Eitape, where a medical orderly

61 G255/754
62 Metzner, Kaewieng to District Officer in Rabaul, 29.5.1914, RKA 2314: 50-51
63 Kopp, 'Dysenterie-Bekämpfung,' 153
64 MB 1910/11: 657
65 MB 1908/09: 394
66 MB 1910/11: 657; 1911/12: 500

was in charge of the hospital, two medical *tultuls* were trained in 1913.[67]

The *Heiltultul* scheme was limited to training men. Rowley noted that in 1913 an experiment with female health assistants was commenced, and the women were to promote the health of nursing mothers and babies.[68] This information may well rest on a mistranslation of the original German text. The scheme mentioned (the training of German women at the Colonial School for Women for work in the colonies) was for the support of white women, not native women.[69] A proposal to train native women in well controlled districts was first made in 1914 by Dr Kersten as part of his submission on the development of health services in the south-east of the Gazelle Peninsula and the Duke of York group. The women's training, for at least one year, would focus on obstetric and baby care.[70] This proposal took into account the difficulty of treating native women in general, but in particular by men. Difficult obstetric cases in native hospitals—some ending in maternal or infant death, or both—had shown that childbirth was not always easy and problem-free for native women as had been lightly assumed in the past.[71] Doctors also found repeatedly that men and boys could be examined readily in a village health survey, but not women. It is perhaps to their credit that they decided that discretion was the better part of medicine. Dr Hoffmann's experience in mid-1912, accompanying the district officer on the tax collection trip to villages around Kaewieng and some 100 kilometres south along the east coast, illustrated the difficulties doctors encountered. This was a district from which many women had been recruited and therefore were unavoidably familiar with western medicine. Rumours began to spread that everybody would be examined for venereal infection; the men did not bring their wives, and Hoffmann

---

67 Draft AR 1913/14: 95

68 Rowley, 'The Promotion of Native Health in German New Guinea,' *South Pacific* 9.5(1957): 393 (quoting from the *Report on the Territory of New Guinea, 1921-2*: 40, in which reference is made to a text in *Amtsblatt* 1913: 139-40). In this he probably followed Reed, *The Making of Modern New Guinea*, 151. It is to be noted that around 1912 Dr Rodenwaldt began training native women as midwives in Togo, making him the founder of the first school for midwives in Africa. Jusatz, *Wandlungen*, 236.

69 The *Koloniale Frauenbund* (Colonial Women's League) opened a training school for women in Bad Weilbach (near Wiesbaden) in 1911. Wives or fiancees of prospective settlers, and also women "from educated families" who wanted to work in the colonies as mothers' companions or nannies were encouraged to attend this school before going there. *Amtsblatt* 1913: 139-40. A second school with a similar aim was set up in 1911 in Carthaus (near Trier). *Kolonie und Heimat* 52(1912/13): 8

70 Kersten, Zur Frage des Bevölkerungsrückganges in Neupommern,' ASTH 19(1915): 576

71 MB 1908/09: 402-3; also Born RKA 2311: 62 f.

accepted that "a medical examination of women was absolutely out of the question as the people's feelings had to be considered and no compulsion was possible in these matters."[72] It is also an indication of how fragile the relationship still was between doctors and villagers. Doctors could not take risks and act in any way likely to impair a precarious rapport.

An immediate change of attitude of the native people was noted when arsphenamines (Salvarsan and Neosalvarsan) were used for the treatment of yaws. Even the most severe yaws healed rapidly following a short course of treatment. The results were dramatic and were reported as contributing greatly to creating trust in European doctors and healing methods, so much so that natives suffering from yaws began to seek medical aid without pressure, even people from remote areas with very little contact with whites.[73] While not wanting to disparage the impact and effectiveness of the new treatment, we nevertheless cannot be as sure as the doctors were at the time that it created trust in the medical service in general. Perhaps it merely encouraged patients to seek treatment for a particular complaint for which a miraculous cure was available.

POPULATION DECLINE

Numerous deaths among labourers in Kaiser-Wilhelmsland, outbreaks of dysentery and influenza which caused many deaths in native villages, and the smallpox epidemic which had spread into unknown territories, were signals for alarm and, together with inter-tribal feuds and the small number of children seen in villages, were seen as indications already during the company period that the population was decreasing. There was much speculation on the reasons, but few facts.

In its 1896/7 *Annual Report* the company pointed to "...the adverse effect of feuds on population numbers and low birth rates..."[74] as major reasons for low numbers. These factors dominated thinking for many years whenever the population question arose: much of the blame for population decline and health problems was put on the native population itself. Doctors, faced with

---

72 Hoffmann, 'Ueber die Gesundheitsverhältnisse der Eingeborenen im nördlichen Neu-mecklenburg,' *Amtsblatt* 5(1913): 115

73 MB 1912/13: 52; quarterly report 1.7.–31.10.1912, RKA 5772: 196-7; Kersten, 'Zur Frage des Bevölkerungsrückganges', 566. Arsphenamines were discovered by Ehrlich in 1909.

74 AR 1896-7: 133

medical evidence, gradually lost confidence in this theory, but planters used this explanation to the last days of German rule. So, for instance, the New Guinea Company which in a submission to the Colonial Office dated 29 July 1914, in which the proposed labour ordinance was discussed, reiterated yet again, that the government should create peace and order among natives by ending intertribal feuds, and put an end to birth control, both measures which would prevent a further population decline.[75]

To put an end to such customary practices became a preoccupation. Intertribal feuding was seen as the easiest problem to tackle because it was the most conspicuous. Whether feuds had the impact on population growth that observers assumed is another question. Typical was a report of a skirmish observed by missionaries in Bogadjim, when there were several wounded and one death;[76] hardly a great impact on population. Equally typical was Parkinson's assertion that shortly before his visit to the north coast of New Britain, inland tribes had attacked coastal villages and at least one hundred people had died in the fighting.[77] Whatever the accuracy of such reports, they suggested that feuds were constant and deaths were many, but their demographic impact was not known. However, steps taken by the government to settle "incessant feuds among natives" also ended with killings. As districts were "pacified" and opened for recruitment, punitive expeditions claimed victims, as did the last such expedition in the south of Bougainville at the end of 1913 when "the main culprits were shot dead by the troop."[78] But there was comfort in the generally held view that, thanks to government intervention and the civilising influence of missions, feuds were becoming increasingly rare.[79]

Low birth rates were a more difficult problem. The small number of children in New Guinea villages puzzled settlers from the earliest days.[80] Missionary Hoffmann, among others, wondered why families in Bogadjim usually had only two or three children, and often only one, and discovered to his horror that infanticide was practised.[81] Without investigating possible

75 RKA 2314: 8 ff
76 Hoffmann, *Barmer Missionsblatt* 1896: 90-93
77 Parkinson, *Dreissig Jahre in der Südsee* (Stuttgart: Strecker & Schröder, 1907) 208
78 Draft AR 1913/14: 71
79 Neuhauss, *Deutsch Neu-Guinea* (Berlin, Dietrich Reimer, 1911) 133
80 When surveying coastal districts in Kaiser-Wilhelmsland to find a suitable centre for missionary activities, Eich from the Rhenish Mission found the small number of children "striking". *Rheinische Missions-Berichte*, 1888: 55
81 *Rheinische Missions-Berichte*, 1897: 103

reasons, or establishing whether it was as frequent as was assumed, missionaries condemned the practice.[82] A careful population count by missionaries over a period of nearly nine years revealed that the population in the villages of Bongu, Bogadjim (south of the Gogol River), Siar and Ragetta (around Friedrich-Wilhelmshafen), had increased by only five; in other coastal villages known to missionaries, the situation was thought to be similar, and in some nearby mountain villages the population was believed to have fallen by about half. The reasons for this poor growth, or even decline, were seen by missionaries to be birth control and infanticide, centuries of inbreeding and venereal disease, and the complete disregard of hygienic principles.[83]

If there was one point of agreement between missionaries, administration, and planters, it was the need to eradicate practices and customs that reduced the population. Missions took this stand on moral grounds; the administration and planters on economic grounds. Moral exhortation and legal intervention were both tried, but birth control was difficult to prove even for missionaries who had closer contact with villagers than did government officials. Keen to punish offenders, the Divine Word Mission in Monumbo (Potsdamhafen) took it upon itself to intervene directly when it suspected a woman of infanticide, and burnt down her hut, a "mild measure" by mission standards.[84] The mission continued its zealous crusade against women accused of abortion or infanticide and insisted on their arrest and trial, actions which provoked serious unrest.[85] Whether the mission extirpated such practices is doubtful, despite some good press.[86] Dr Liesegang noted that the number of children along the coast of Kaiser-Wilhelmsland was as small as ever. He professed some sympathy for women, "much plagued drudges" who, because of their hard life, had little inclination to bear many children so that contraception and abortion remained common everywhere. He agreed that, in order to promote population growth, intervention was necessary, but foresaw great difficulty as people were not interested in changing their ways. When he tried to discover

---

82 Infanticide is mentioned repeatedly by missionaries, for instance, *Rheinische Missions-Berichte*, 1904: 230; *Gott will es!* 1907: 112; 1912: 25; *Die Katholischen Missionen* 32(1903): 102; also *DKB* 11(1900): 558

83 *Rheinische Missions-Berichte*, 1904: 230 ff – report on a meeting by missionaries to discuss the problems of population decline.

84 Scholz report to Governor, 30.3.1910: RKA 2994: 16 ff

85 See Firth, *New Guinea* 97

86 Neuhauss, a medical doctor who spent about a year in KWL for private studies, asserted in his book that the moral influence of the mission had brought about great improvements, and abortions, infanticide and mutual killings had just about ceased and the population was beginning to increase. Neuhauss 133

the ways and means of contraception and abortion, "people simply smiled but did not answer, although they knew very well what he wanted to know."[87] Even after nearly thirty years of exposure to European influences, such secrets were not given away readily. It is also an indication of how little Germans understood New Guinean people and their culture. More curious still, Liesegang did not connect low fertility with malaria. In the Bismarck Archipelago birth control was also believed to affect population size. Infanticide was reported particularly in western New Britain and in New Ireland, but less so on the Gazelle Peninsula.[88]

Emphasising birth control was a very convenient way of looking at the problem; it absolved colonists from any criticism, but provoked outbursts of moral rectitude which may well have led to overestimating its incidence. Little attempt was made to understand why natives took measures to control the number of children other than concluding that natives were too lazy to raise large families.[89] Laziness, in the eyes of the colonisers, was a distinct moral failing. This superficial assessment ignored deep cultural differences in values: New Guineans maintained a precarious population balance, but Germans promoted population growth.

While it could not be known why there were so few children when the Germans first arrived in New Guinea, latching on to birth control as the explanation is understandable, for Germans were used to large families, especially in rural regions.[90] Yet, when research shed new light on the question, and Koch concluded that malaria was a cause of high infant mortality[91]—an insight surely crucial to understanding New Guinean demographics—the findings were ignored for years. This was so not only in New Guinea, but also in Germany. As late as 1910, Matthias Erzberger, from the Centre Party, who had made colonies his speciality, sensationalised the issue in the Reichstag. "Everywhere there would be plenty of children, if not so many young and germinating lives fell victim to their savage unnatural parents" he thundered,

---

87   MB 1910/11: 657; 1911/12: 501

88   Parkinson, 'Dreissig Jahre in der Südsee' 71; 208-9; 267. (On the other hand, Parkinson noted (483) that on Buka and Bougainville, where infanticide was rare, large families were not uncommon, and the population was maintaining itself.

89   A view summed up by Neuhauss, Neu Guinea, 131: "Papuans are lazy and do not work more than absolutely necessary for survival. If they had large families, they would have to clear forests for larger plantations. This costs a lot of sweat and therefore they ensure in good time that the family does not become too large."

90   The birth rate in Germany before 1914 was 4.5 children per woman. Külz, 'Zur Biologie und Pathologie des Nachwuchses bei den Naturvölkern', ASTH 23(1919). Beiheft 3: 75

91   Koch's address to the Colonial Council, DKB 11(1900): 947

when the protection of indigenous peoples was discussed in the Reichstag budget debates.[92] While birth control, blood feuds and racial degeneration were uppermost in the thinking of Germans as the causes of population decline—that is, as long as responsibility could be laid squarely on New Guineans—there was little incentive to look for other causes. Dempwolff's observation that Europeans readily assumed that contraception or infanticide were the reasons for the small number of children and population decline, when in fact the low birth rate was due to disease,[93] was also ignored by missionaries and planters, and doctors only began to take notice of it much later. Dr Hoffmann did so in 1912—after eight years' work in Friedrich-Wilhelmshafen and three in Kaewieng he was one of the most experienced practitioners in dealing with malaria. He argued that the high incidence of malaria among villagers in Kaewieng suggested that malaria was introduced not long before, and had led to high infant mortality and, in all probability, also caused many spontaneous abortions.[94] He had gone one step further and implicated malaria not only in high infant mortality but also as an abortifacient, a point seemingly not noted by his colleagues.

With eugenic theories on population decline promoted in Germany, it was not surprising that they should find an echo in New Guinea, particularly in relation to reproduction. The idea that inbreeding because of the isolation of the tribal groups led to degeneration, which manifested itself in low birth rates, became firmly established, as did the notion of the "physical vitality" of a people. Richard Parkinson, who had lived on the Gazelle Peninsula since 1882, and had extensively studied the people of the Bismarck Archipelago, observed that "a certain weariness with life [robbed] the population of its vitality" and had led to a gradual population decline already before the arrival of whites.[95] Dr Stephan, a naval doctor who spent a year on the survey ship *Möwe* in 1904, and returned in 1907 as leader of a German Naval expedition, inferred from his observations in central and southern New Ireland that the only reason for low birth rates was centuries of inbreeding which had led to a kind of degeneration, an "exhaustion of the procreative capacities" of the tribes. He found that on average a couple had only two children; five was the highest number he came across.[96] As he described four to five children as a "moderate" number, two

---

92 He called them *wilde Rabeneltern. Steno-graphische Berichte der Verhandlungen des Reichstags,* 1909/10, (12. Legislaturperiode, 2. Session, 31.1.1910) vol. 259: 928

93 Dempwolff, 'Aussterbende Völker' 413

94 Hoffmann report on population in Kaewieng district and north-east coast of New Ireland, July 1912. *Amtsblatt* 1913: 119

95 Parkinson, *Dreissig Jahre in der Südsee* 267

96 Stephan, report to Governor, 11 Nov. 1908, RKA 2311: 138 ff

children were well below his norm. Dr Born, who spent two rain-sodden months in central New Ireland to examine the population, also concluded that inbreeding was one reason for population decline, but he was not as pessimistic about the long term prospects as Stephan. Born was convinced that, as pacification brought much greater contact between clans, this would also bring new vigour and vitality to the population.[97] A conspicuous population feature was high masculinity and it was regarded as "a sign of racial degeneration."[98]

Regardless of how much emphasis was put on birth control, blood feuds and degeneration, it was obvious that these factors alone did not fully explain population decline, particularly not in New Ireland, a recruiting ground for men and women since the early 1880s. Recruitment and its effect on population numbers became the central question in a long struggle between the administration and planters that began in 1906 when the government proposed a ban on recruitment of women from northern and central New Ireland. The question is explored in detail by Firth in the chapter 'Depopulation and the Planters' in his *New Guinea under the Germans*[99] and there is no need to repeat the all-important political and economic aspects of the question. Instead, I propose to concentrate on some public health issues that came to the fore as a result of the many reports written by doctors and district officers in response to Governor Hahl's requests for information.

Doctors were unanimous on the close connection between recruitment and venereal infection, but less so on the effect of venereal disease on population numbers. Theoretically venereal diseases should not have been a problem, as examination of indentured labourers was compulsory so as to prevent their returning home with an infection. In practice the spread was not controlled quite so readily. Infections were not always completely healed when treatment was completed; men and women went on home leave without a medical check, and it was not unknown for employers to send sick labourers home so as to save on hospital costs.[100] Drs Born and Runge, both writing about New Ireland, were most emphatic that venereal disease had a detrimental effect on population growth, mainly because it caused sterility in women. In central New Ireland, where in each village visited by Born a number of men and women had worked as plantation labourers, he found gonorrhoea

---

97 Born report 8.7.1908, RKA 2311: 69
98 MB 1911/12: 505. Also Fülleborn report III, 1908 quoted in Fischer, *Die Hamburger Südsee-Expedition*: 44. Fülleborn was the leader of the Hamburg Expedition to the South Sea (1908-10) for the first year of the expedition.
99 Firth, *New Guinea*, chapter 6, 112-135
100 Hoffmann, 21.10.1907, RKA 2310: 90 ff

and venereal granuloma to be widespread, and he recommended that systematic examination and treatment for venereal infection should be introduced in villages.[101] Quite a different opinion was expressed by Dr Siebert a short time later.[102] A check in villages along the north east coast of New Ireland revealed only one case of gonorrhoea and two cases of suspected syphilis; in the immediate vicinity of Kaewieng the incidence of gonorrhoea was much higher. But Siebert had a different perspective: he compared the incidence of venereal infection in New Ireland with that in Java, where it was much higher. As the high level of venereal disease did not seem to affect population growth in Java, Siebert was confident that its effect on population size in New Ireland was exaggerated.[103] Hoffmann was clearly influenced by Siebert's view and concluded that, much as venereal infection merited attention, too great an emphasis on it tended to detract from other important health issues. In particular it fostered a belief that by combating venereal disease, the most important native health problems were being solved.[104]

Governor Hahl presented his views on the population question to the Colonial Office and recommended increased medical services as the solution. In his submission he argued that the decline in New Ireland was due first to degeneration which was the result of continuous inbreeding, second to the lack of women of child-bearing age because of recruiting, and last to diseases that affected the population, that is, respiratory tract infections, dysentery, malaria, whooping cough, venereal infections, tropical ulcers and skin diseases.[105] He made the point that pacification, which led to much wider contact among the population, was taking care of degeneration. A first step therefore would be to ban recruitment of women but, for political reasons, it was a measure to be taken only for very limited periods and discrete regions. This left a medical solution as the only practicable way of dealing with the problem. In his opinion the population could only become healthy and be able to produce more children if the various health disorders were being medically treated. For such an undertaking greatly expanded medical services were essential.

With medical services as the chief weapon to combat population decline,

101 Born, RKA 2311: 68; Runge, RKA 2311: 77
102 As a member of Prof. Neisser's syphilis survey team in Batavia, Dr Siebert had spent six months examining skin and venereal diseases in Batavia. Before returning to Germany, he spent two months in northern New Ireland in 1908 where he accompanied the medical officer and the district officer on a number of trips and surveyed the population.
103 K. Siebert, 'Ueber Wesen und Verbreitung von Haut- und Geschlechtskrankheiten in Nord-Neumecklenburg,' *ASTH* 13 (1909): 201-14
104 Hoffmann, 'Gesundheitsverhältnisse im nördlichen Neumecklenburg,' 121
105 Hahl to RKA 25.10.1908, RKA 2311: 50 ff; also MB 1908/09: 419-20

Hahl proposed a medical service for Namatanai, based in a native hospital. The crucial difference in that service was the role of the doctor. Although he was to be based at that hospital, he was to work as a "travelling doctor" (*Wanderarzt*) who would go out the villages and work there, rather than patients being brought to him.[106] This was a new departure: on other stations medical services were set up to care for the labour force, and villagers came second; under the new proposal the travelling doctor's central concern was to be the villagers. The Namatanai medical service came into operation in October 1911, when Dr Kröning took up work. However, as the hospital catered also for labourers from surrounding plantations, his duties at the hospital took up quite some time, and in practice as much of his time was spent in hospital as in villages.

The need for a travelling doctor had been pointed out by Dr Born in his report on his trip to central New Ireland.[107] When he spent a few days in each of a number of villages along the coast, people came to him and, when necessary, even stayed overnight in small huts built to serve as make-shift hospitals. This convinced him that a travelling doctor would be the best way to bring medical services to villagers. He was supported by Dr Wick who was working at the native hospital in Rabaul. Wick was also keen to get medical services into villages, but much needed trips into the wider surroundings of Rabaul to gain the confidence of the villagers had to take second place to work at the hospital.[108] Despite repeated recommendations, it was 1914 before money was allocated specifically for a travelling doctor.

What Hahl omitted to recommend for improving health in New Ireland is as important as his recommendations. He stressed the need for more medical services and hospitals as the first line of attack on diseases in the indigenous population. Preoccupied with the effects of venereal diseases and respiratory tract infections, he did not mention public works like sanitation or the provision of clean water, despite the fact that dysentery was "the scourge of the people". Yet, clean water as a cheap way of improving health had been part of Dr Wendland's recommendations to the governor. Malaria barely rated a mention, nor did public works to eradicate mosquito breeding grounds, abundant in the Namatanai district.[109] As far as the governor was concerned, therapeutics was the way to a healthy population.

---

106 Hahl to RKA 25.10.1908, RKA 2311: 53
107 Born 'Die Gesundheitsverhältnisse der Eingeborenen im mittleren Neu-Mecklenburg' [report on health conditions of natives in central New Ireland] of 29.7.1908, RKA 2311: 55-73
108 MB 1908/09: 366
109 RKA 2311: 50-56; 135

Külz Report

In the two years before the outbreak of war the population question prompted a number of medical surveys, so that by mid-1914 there was a good picture of the health situation in most districts under government control. The Australian authorities seem to have used only the 1913 report by Dr Kopp which dealt with the north coast of New Britain.[110] Other reports might have been of interest also, foremost those of Dr Külz. Although most of the reports submitted by doctors[111] reflect views espoused by Külz for years, his reports throw into relief the state of native health in the colony at the outbreak of war, and so I discuss them in some detail.

As noted before, it was intended that Külz be appointed Chief Medical Officer for German New Guinea; he arrived in Rabaul in October 1913. On the premise that New Guineans had to be healthy and fit to work on plantations and contribute their share to the development of the colonial economy, and at the same time grow in numbers, Külz's task was to develop and coordinate a health system to achieve these ends. But before taking up his appointment, together with Dr Leber, an eye specialist, he was charged with carrying out a health survey of the whole of German New Guinea, which included addressing the problems of population growth.[112]

Külz realised that there was not enough demographic data to corroborate long held views that the population was declining, but believed that this was so in districts under European influence. However, the central question for

110 Translated and published by the British Administration of German New Guinea as 'The native Population of New Britain: do they decline? and what are the causes', in the Rabaul *Government Gazette*, 1(5) 15.12.1914, and 2(1) 15.1.1915

111 Other reports published by doctors on native health in the last years before war in the *Amtsblatt* were: W. Hoffmann, 'Ueber die Gesundheitsverhältnisse der Eingeborenen im nordöstlichen Neumecklenburg', *Amtsblatt* 5(1913): 114-31; Kersten, 'Bericht über die Expedition nach Morobe,' *Amtsblatt* 5(1913): 131-2; 'Die Sulka Siedlungen am St. Georgskanal,' *Amtsblatt* 6(1914): 213-7; ' W. Wick, 'Die gesundheitlichen Verhältnisse im mittleren Neumecklenburg,' *Amtsblatt* 3(1911): 234-5; 240-1; 'Besuch der Witu-Inseln', *Amtsblatt* 6(1914): 180-1. Other reports published around the same time were less readily accessible to the Australian authorities, such as Börnstein's medical and ethnographic surveys of the Willaumez Peninsula in *DKB* 25(1914): 828-32, and of Manus (*DKB* 26(1915): 154-61

112 The team of Külz and Leber operated under the title *Medizinisch-Demographische Deutsch Neuguinea-Expedition des Reichs-Kolonialamts* [Medico-demographic German New Guinea research expedition sponsored by the Colonial Office]. Under the terms of agreement, all reports of the expedition had to be published under joint names, although both Külz and Leber undertook separate research. For example, on the Gazelle Peninsula, Külz undertook the research and wrote the report; Leber went to Bougainville and Buka, but his report on that research trip was not published; it remained with the Australian authorities and is now in the Australian Archives (Victoria), MP 367, File No. 404/11/52. Leber was on his way back to Germany when war broke out and he spent the war years in the Dutch East Indies.

him was less that of decline than the potential for population growth, whether and how a downward trend could be reversed. Therefore he set out to establish birth rates as indicators of the potential for population growth. Low birth rates would indicate that the population was not replacing itself. Alternatively, birth rates could be such that the population maintained itself at a given size. The preferred possibility was that birth rates were high enough to stimulate population growth with appropriate health care measures. In order to establish crude birth rates he developed a sample technique for counting populations whose concepts of time differed from European norms, and among whom age was difficult to determine, unless the people happened to live in an area where missionaries kept records. He worked on the principle that women, despite their low cultural level, were intelligent and remembered the number of children they had borne, and that they would be willing to talk about it if they were spoken to in a reasonable manner.[113] From this premise he proceeded by asking a number of women questions on their child-bearing history, making a clear distinction between women past child-bearing age and those younger. The figures to be established from both groups were the number of children a woman had borne and the number who had died. In the latter category, a distinction had to be made between those who died before the age of one, and later deaths, with age one deemed to be the time a child began to walk. The number of stillbirths was difficult to establish, as it was impossible to know whether women distinguished between abortions, stillbirths and neonatal deaths, but was important to establish fecundity. The number of children born, less the number of children who died, gave the 'net figure growing up'. Other figures to be calculated were the proportion of children to adults, and the proportion of the sexes.

Külz examined the population of five villages south-west of Herbertshöhe,[114] four villages east of Kabanga Bay,[115] six villages southwest of Cape Gazelle,[116] and several hamlets in the Toma district. He drew up a chart for each individual with all health details. In this way he established health profiles for all the villages examined, a useful data base for follow-up work. The

---

113 A premise which would have been disputed by some of today's demographers. See for instance, Lea and Lewis, 'Masculinity in Papua New Guinea', in Kosinski and Webb, *Population at Microscale*, (New Zealand Geographical Society, 1976) 65 ff

114 L. Külz and A. Leber, 'Bericht der medizinisch-demographischen Südsee-Expedition über die Gazellehalbinsel,' *DKB* 25(1914,) 782-89. The villages were Tukabar, Bitagalip, Ramale, Livuan and Ulakun

115 The villages were Nanalar, Burbur, Karu and Kabanga

116 The villages were Ballada, Katakotoi, Tabunu, Ratavul, Togoro and Tavui

figures for the Gazelle Peninsula from a sample of 471 women showed that fertility rates were high, with an average of 5.5 live births per woman; the number of sterile women was low; abortion was practised but without apparently affecting later fertility. He estimated from figures given to him by the Catholic priests (who apparently had gained the confidence of their parishioners to the extent that they were told of abortions) that there was one abortion for every five live births, but suspected that the number was likely to be higher. Infant and child mortality was high at 52 per cent. The first year rate was not exceptionally high at 29 per cent, a figure similar to that obtaining in Germany not many decades earlier, and still valid in some Prussian provinces.[117] But mortality was high in the age groups past the first year and it was not possible to establish causes of death other than a broad distinction between internal and external causes. Malaria was the most obvious cause, but its effect varied greatly throughout the Gazelle Peninsula, with very low mortality in the malaria-free Toma district. He speculated that once children began to walk, they were exposed to minor injuries to the feet and legs which rapidly led to ulcers and often ended fatally. The high masculinity with 122 boys to 100 girls puzzled him; in 1914 he speculated that girls were much more likely to be victims of infanticide as they were regarded as less valuable to the defence of the tribe. This practice might give rise to a tendency to produce more men.[118] On further reflection he was not satisfied with that explanation— it was a question to be solved in the future,[119] but he was mindful that it had an effect on population numbers.[120]

A visit to the Sulka people indicated that conditions varied a great deal on the Gazelle Peninsula. A section of the Sulka people, some 1100, were resettled by the government in 1908/9 because of the constant attacks on them by the Gakhais.[121] There was a mission station near their new settlement in Mope and missionaries kept a close eye on them. Under the period of observation and record keeping, there was certainly a higher death than birth rate. A very high rate of pneumonia deaths suggested that a vicious circle had been set in motion: the labour force that used to be available to maintain houses and plantations was no longer available, partly because of recruiting and partly because some had returned to their old settlement; this affected nutrition in quality and quantity which in turn affected the people's resistance to acute and chronic infections. The ensuing high mortality increased the fear of spirits in

117 Külz 'Biologie und Pathologie' 123
118 Külz and Leber, 784-86
119 Külz, 'Biologie und Pathologie' 80

120 L. Külz, Ueber das Aussterben der Natur-völker. *Archiv für Frauenkunde und Eugenik* 52/3(1919): 142-3
121 *Amtsblatt* 1910: 56

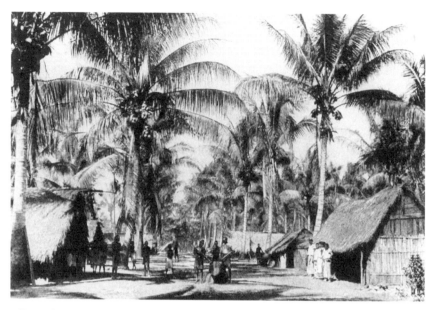

Village of Tobera on the Gazelle Peninsula

a superstitious people who then moved their huts to avoid the alleged enemy. The new houses were not built with the same care as the old ones because of the lack of labour and they no longer provided sufficient shelter from strong winds and heavy rains. An examination revealed that the Sulka had a much poorer state of health than the other groups examined. Of eighty-one men 37 per cent reacted positively to tuberculosis tests, as did 24 per cent of the women and children. Clinical tuberculosis was diagnosed in several cases, some in an advanced stage. Malaria incidence was high; 61 per cent of the children at the mission school had enlarged spleens. Tinea, yaws, and conjunctivitis were at the same rate as in the remainder of the Gazelle Peninsula population, but there was no venereal disease among the men examined. A sample of thirty women still in their reproductive years showed that they had borne 118 children, not a bad fertility rate. Nutrition appeared to be poor and so was the water supply.[122] The experience of the Sulka resettlement because of intertribal feuds puts the government's efforts to protect a population group very much in question. Some may well have been saved from slaughter by

122 Külz and Leber, 787-8

their traditional foe, yet many succumbed to diseases brought about by dislocation. The most damning evidence is their much poorer overall health than that of the Gazelle population as a whole.

In his overall assessment of health of the Gazelle Peninsula population, Külz's first point was that the notion of the population declining because of blood feuds, inbreeding, abortions and infanticide was utterly fallacious for, if this were the case, the population would have declined well and truly before the arrival of Europeans. What was needed in all villages was basic hygiene and medical services. Basic hygiene would improve health in general, and medical services would ensure that the prevalent diseases were brought under control. With an average of 5.5 live births per woman of which on average 2.6 children reached adulthood, particular attention had to be paid to infants and children; by keeping them alive and healthy, the population would increase quickly.[123]

In the villages surveyed, Külz found very much the same problems as others had before him: venereal disease—usually gonorrhoea or venereal granuloma, and some rare cases of syphilis—was present in and around Herbertshöhe and Rabaul, and certainly needed attention. Hookworm was widespread; while not dangerous in itself, he argued that in combination with malaria a high degree of infection affected a child's development. Yaws was also widespread, as were goitres in certain areas. The diet was satisfactory and villages were kept clean, unlike the people themselves; in particular the clothing forced on them was in a filthy state. In many villages there was no water and it had to be brought in from a long way; others had an insufficient supply of poor quality water. The high number of eye diseases which, until their exact nature was established with further research, were called "suppurating conjunctivitis" were grounds for particular comment. Eleven women out of 471 were blind in one eye, and five completely blind.[124]

In Kaiser-Wilhelmsland Külz found his research more difficult. In districts without missionary influence, people lacked any understanding of what a doctor was about, and he had to spend much time proving his credentials. His findings from samples in the Morobe district, among the Kai people in the Finschhafen district, and in Eitape again showed that fertility was high with an average of 4.9 children for women past child-bearing age.[125] While infant

123 Külz and Leber: 786-7; Külz, 'Biologie und Pathologie' 124
124 Külz and Leber, 784
125 Külz, 'Biologie und Pathologie' 127-133

mortality up to the age of one was relatively low (15 per cent in the Morobe samples, 22 per cent in Eitape), it was much higher after that age, giving total infant mortality rates of 37 per cent in the Morobe samples, 46 per cent in Finschhafen, and 43 per cent in Eitape. Despite high infant mortality, there were enough children left to ensure a steady population.

In northern New Ireland the situation differed greatly. A sample of 154 women (past child-bearing age) had borne 394 children. With an infant mortality rate of 35 per cent, a woman raised on average 1.7 children. This low figure clearly indicated that the population was declining. Külz ascribed this in no uncertain terms to the consequences of excessive recruitment, especially that of women, and argued that up to 1909, when mainly single women were recruited from New Ireland, their recruitment had been a form of prostitution; the situation had not improved much when married women only could be recruited; venereal infection had spread widely despite medical treatment. In his sample 22 per cent of the women were sterile, usually as a result of gonorrhoea. In a population in which the number of women was smaller than men, such infertility certainly affected population size. The close connection between recruitment and number of children was also demonstrated when it was found that of 220 married couples, those in which neither partner had been recruited had nearly twice as many children as those where one or both partners had been away on plantation work.[126] Külz's research confirmed the devastating effect of recruitment on population numbers. Medical intervention alone was not going to halt population decline.

In Külz's view, one potentially serious disease was tuberculosis, and testing the level of infection with the von Pirquet method was an important part of his examinations. He found that rates differed, with the highest incidence of positive reactions in New Ireland.[127] Of 247 men tested, 44 per cent reacted positively, as did 30 per cent of the women and 9 per cent of children. Labourers from New Ireland working in Eitape showed an even higher rate, with 54 per cent testing positively. Among the sample of forty-nine coastal people in the Eitape district, 20 per cent had a positive reaction; of the ten men with a positive reaction seven had worked on European plantations. In a group of sixty-two men who had just arrived from the hinterland of Eitape, only one had a positive reaction; he was the only one to

126 Külz, 'Biologie und Pathologie' 59, 123, 171-2
127 Külz, 'Biologie und Pathologie' 148. He did not state where in New Ireland he did his research, but indications are that he arrived in Kaewieng just before war broke out, so that he did not have a chance to go to central or southern New Ireland.

have worked on a plantation; all others were recruited for the first time.[128]

These test results, together with those obtained by Kopp on the north coast of New Britain late in 1912,[129] and by Kersten early in 1913 in Morobe, Bogadjim and the native hospital in Friedrich-Wilhelmshafen,[130] convinced Külz that the introduction of tuberculosis was recent, that is since European settlement in New Guinea, with Europeans as the main source of infection. Whereas other doctors wondered about the rapid course of the disease, he was sure that it was so virulent and led to death quickly because the first infection was in adults; there was no exposure to the disease in childhood as was common in Europe and hence no opportunity to develop immunity.[131] In his opinion tuberculosis had nearly reached the point where it would turn from an acute infectious to an endemic disease and as such become a serious public health problem,[132] but while he urged that this must be prevented, he never spelt out how. By the time he arrived in New Guinea, the practice of sending home native tuberculosis patients not in an advanced stage and showing few clinical symptoms,[133] was well established, and contributed to the spread of the infection. The most striking example of how tuberculosis spread came from Taminugetu, a village on the south side of the Huon Peninsula. In 1898 a young man returned after working in Herbertshöhe for some time with symptoms of lung disease (observed by missionaries). Over the next few years some of his relatives died with similar symptoms. When Külz tested a sample of ten young men, seven were infected, and one showed

128 Külz, 'Biologie und Pathologie' 148. Wigley ('Tuberculosis and New Guinea' 172-73) put forward that German doctors inoculated with tuberculin for tuberculosis in 1912. In the translation of the Annual Reports by Sack & Clark the term 'immunised' is also used. (AR 1912/13: 360) This may rest on a misunderstanding of the word *'impfen'* which normally means 'inoculation' or 'vaccination'. However, German doctors also used the term when describing tuberculosis testing with the von Pirquet method. It is clear from the context that they were testing for tuberculosis, not inoculating against it. However, Kersten reported from Friedrich-Wilhelmshafen that he attempted tuberculin therapy in two cases. Quarterly Report 1.4.-30.6.1913, RKA 5772: 246

129 Kopp, 'Bevölkerungsrückgang' 729-50.

130 Kersten, 'Die Tuberkulose in Kaiser-Wilhelms-Land,' *ASTH* 19(1915): 101-8. The results from the Morobe district were interesting, as they confirmed yet again the close connection between plantation labour and tuberculosis. A group of men from villages on the upper Waria all tested negatively (men only tested); on the lower Waria women and children tested negatively, but 23% of men were positive. In Morobe the result was similar, with women and children testing negatively, and 27 % of men positively. In Bogadjim there were positive reactions in all groups: 8% of children aged 6-14, 20% of women, and 27 % of men.

131 Külz, 'Biologie und Pathologie' 149

132 ibid. 154

133 MB 1906/07: 203; 1907/08: 417

clinical symptoms.[134] With tuberculosis infected Europeans dying in all centres and in all occupational groups—missionaries, planters and traders—infection was possible through various kinds of contact. It had certainly spread to remote parts; Dr Bürgers diagnosed one advanced case of tuberculosis in 1914 in a village on the May River, a tributary of the Sepik.[135]

Külz also brought the focus back onto malaria, which he considered the greatest enemy of health, affecting people throughout their lives. It caused directly many infant deaths, but, he argued, as it was likely that the weakest died, it could be regarded as a kind of selection process which eliminated weaklings. As more insidious he regarded the effects of repeated malaria attacks on the overall health of even the strongest survivor. Because of anaemia as a result of malaria, many children remained sickly for years, and it seriously weakened resistance to other diseases, particularly intestinal infections. Long lactation, frowned upon by many doctors as it tended to act as a contraceptive, was to be encouraged, as the best means of preventing intestinal diseases, often fatal in malaria-weakened infants. With a child-bearing period of about twenty-five years, native women were able to produce a sizeable number of children, even with long lactation.[136]

Külz's reports indicated that the focus of health care in villages should be on infants and children, a point reinforced in his later articles. This entailed care of mothers, for healthy children could not be born and raised by sick mothers. To this end women had to be protected, and their work load reduced, so that their time could be devoted to their families. Recruitment for work outside the district was socially disruptive and detrimental to health, a harmful practice that had to be stopped.[137] While advocating pro-natalist policies, he realised that raising a large number of children would have an effect on women, but his concern was solely because of the adverse effects existing work practices had on their capacity to bear and raise a large number of healthy children. He was not so much interested in bettering the lives of women as in redirecting them. Possible social consequences as a result of a sudden population increase did not come into his calculations. Rational economic development demanded intervention to bring about fundamental changes in the New Guinean society and, given the opportunity, he was not reluctant to intervene.

Perhaps the most striking aspect of Külz's reports is the underlying assump-

134 Külz, 'Biologie und Pathologie' 149
135 Bürgers' report on the Sepik River Expedition, 20.2.1914, RKA 5773: 63
136 Külz, 'Biologie und Pathologie 30, 140-1
137 Külz, 'Biologie und Pathologie' 61

tion that New Guineans would fall in readily with his prescriptions, or that their and the colonists' interests coincided. It was not a question of what the people wanted or needed from their point of view, but of ensuring that they met the requirements of a colonial plantation economy. If what was needed was a large labour force, it was up to the women of New Guinea to produce and raise large families. Külz's task in this scheme was the provision of an appropriate medical support system to play its part by caring for the human resources of the future.

When Külz published his articles in 1919 he thought it unlikely that Germany would regain its colonies (certainly not the Pacific colonies), so his recommendations on steps to improve indigenous health were implicit rather than spelt out. Neither had his 1914 article on the Gazelle Peninsula contained any recommendations; it was the first of a series of articles, and the future course of action was to be outlined when the survey was completed. The direction medical services might have taken in New Guinea had the Germans remained there must of course be conjectural, but it is certain that Külz considered hygienic improvements as important as medical services. As Chief Medical Officer, a new position on the New Guinea establishment and of a higher level than previous medical positions, his views and recommendations would have carried weight not only in the colony but also in Berlin. He was after all mandated to improve health and hygiene of the indigenous population.[138] With his views on the effect of recruitment on population numbers, the debate on recruitment would undoubtedly have become even more acrimonious.

As an astute observer Külz highlighted crucial areas of concern, neglected for years. By casting aside popular fallacies on racial degeneration, he was able to see—and enabled others to see—the adverse effects of colonial activities, poor hygiene, endemic diseases and those introduced with the advent of colonialism. He saw clearly that health problems were as much the result of social, economic and environmental conditions as of pathogens.

By the beginning of the second decade, Külz's was not the only voice advocating changes in native health policies. For example, a German Society for the Protection of Indigenous Peoples was founded in 1913,[139] which helped to create a different atmosphere, an awareness that money had to be

138 RKA to Hahl 24.4.1913, RKA 6047: 8

139 Deutsche Gesellschaft für Eingeborenenschutz. *DKZ* 30(1913): 834. The society's objective was the more humane treatment of natives in German colonies. Among its members were people familiar with New Guinea, such as Prof. Krämer, Prof. Neuhauss, Dr Thilenius, and Flierl from the Neuendettelsau Mission; the Rhenish Mission was also a member.

spent if colonies were to become economically viable through the work of a healthy and plentiful population. Reports published by research expeditions to New Guinea also discussed the population question and pointed to the poor state of health of many of the peoples they had visited and the urgent need to stimulate population growth.[140] The population question was not limited to New Guinea, as is evident from a competition sponsored by the Hamburg shipping magnate Eduard Woermann in 1913. The topic of the prize essay, "What are the practical measures to increase birth rates and reduce child mortality in native populations—the economically most valuable assets of our colonies?",[141] pointed to an issue common to all German colonies. Moreover, the colonial population question was not debated in isolation in Germany, for falling birth rates and ways to counter them within Germany were discussed widely in professional and government circles and thereby benefited the discussion on colonial needs.[142]

Changing attitudes were reflected in increased budget allocations for native health by the Reichstag. It is ironic that in the 1914 budget New Guinea 's turn had finally come and increased allocations were made to all hospitals for operating costs and outpatient services, particularly services for villagers.[143] An additional grant of 61,400 Mark was for a new program, the travelling doctor. Two teams consisting each of one doctor, one medical orderly and ten native orderlies, field and medical equipment and medications were financed.[144] The teams were to go into villages to treat people with particular emphasis on worm infestations and yaws. These two conditions were believed

140 For example, G. Friederici, 'Wissenschaftliche Ergebnisse einer amtlichen Forschungsreise nach dem Bismarck-Archipelago im Jahre 1908,' *Mitteilungen aus den Deutschen Schutzgebieten*, 1912, Ergänzungsheft 5: 91. Also, K. Sapper, 'Wissenschaftliche Ergebnisse einer amtlichen Forschungsreise nach dem Bismarck-Archipelago im Jahre 1908,' *Mitteilungen aus den Deutschen Schutzgebieten*, 1910, Ergänzungsheft 3: 102. Sapper was a geographer, Friederici an ethnographer.

141 *DKB* 24(1913): 642-3

142 Külz, 'Ueber das Aussterben' 114

143 From 1907 to 1911 the recurrent annual budget for public health and hospital services (not including salaries for doctors and medical orderlies and capital expenditure) was around 52,000 Mark. Allocation for recurrent costs rose to 98,600 Mark in 1913, and 111,500 Mark in 1914. The total expenditure for health services for the whole of German New Guinea was 8.6% of the 1913 Budget, and 12% of the 1914 Budget. *Etat für das Schutzgebiet Neuguinea 1914* [Budget for German New Guinea 1914].

144 It was probably intended to have one team in the Old Protectorate, and the other in the Island Territory. The sum of 61,400 Mark was calculated as follows: 25,000 Mark for salaries of two doctors and two medical orderlies; 16,000 Mark for their trip to New Guinea and personal equipment; 2,800 Mark for field equipment (tents, fields beds, etc.); 4,600 Mark for wages, food and clothing of native orderlies; 13,000 Mark for medical equipment (instruments, medications, dressings, etc.).

to have a debilitating effect which might render people very susceptible to other infectious diseases such as dysentery and tuberculosis[145] and, surely no small consideration, were conditions for which there was a readily administered remedy available. There is nothing to indicate that provisions specifically for public works in native villages were made in the budget; nevertheless, it is a great pity that there was no chance to test just how much, or how little, native health would have improved with the increased expenditure for medical treatment.

The Germans were confronted with a number of health problems in the native population. One group was diseases regarded as endemic before colonisation: malaria, yaws, skin diseases, ulcers, eye diseases, hookworm, and leprosy. The other was exotic diseases introduced by Europeans; in the main they were crowd infections such as smallpox, dysentery, rubella, mumps, tuberculosis, and venereal disease.

Problems in the first group were handled by the colonial health service with differing degrees of success. Ulcers and skin diseases were the most obvious conditions; as they were so common, the largest number of people were treated and people sought help most readily for them. Hygienic improvements to prevent skin infections depended on changes of personal habits and a water supply, and were therefore much more difficult to effect than treatment with fungicides or parasiticides. It seems that ophthalmology was one field of medicine where doctors were not confident of undertaking other than topical treatment. Eye infections, such as conjunctivitis and trachoma, were treated regularly by doctors, but the first record of surgical intervention was early in 1914.[146] Whether the eye specialist Leber, the second member of the medico-demographic team was sent to New Guinea in 1913 simply to do research and identify 'interesting' eye problems, or to treat people, or to train other doctors in ophthalmic work, is not known from what little information there is on his work.

Successful and simple treatment of yaws was not possible until arsphenamines came on the market. Before these drugs became available, the course of treatment was so demanding of man-hours that the uncertainty of

145 This was the official explanation for introducing a hookworm eradication program. As has been mentioned in the second chapter, ankylostomiasis suddenly was seen as a serious problem when European children were found to be infested. To what extent this discovery contributed to the decision to undertake such a program in native villages remains speculative.

146 Two blind Baining men, never having seen Europeans, but heard about them, agreed to go with Külz to Rabaul, where he successfully restored their sight. Külz and Leber, 784

outcome bore no relation to the amount of time spent on treatment, hence it was attempted only for the most severe cases. The first use of the drugs was made 1912; from then on, because of their efficacy and ease of use, they were used regularly, and were eminently suitable to the work of the travelling doctor. Treatment of hookworm with Thymol became a standard procedure for labourers in hospitals, but no attempt was made to treat or eradicate hookworm in villages until a travelling doctor was available. There is nothing to suggest that sanitary measures were to be implemented at the same time as clearing up the infestation among villagers.

When it came to malaria, the situation was paradoxical indeed. On the one hand, enormous sums were spent in Germany on extensive scientific research and exciting discoveries were made. But at the same time as it was established how the disease was transmitted and how therapy combined with ecological measures could control it, malaria was spread through colonial activities into previously uninfested places. There was little relationship between research in Germany and practical needs in New Guinea once field work there had established the complexities and high cost of malaria eradication.

Exotic diseases presented different problems. Of the acute crowd infections, smallpox and cholera were brought under control and did not recur. Cholera outbreaks were prevented with quarantine measures, and smallpox with vaccination, undoubtedly the most effective public health program undertaken, in as much as it prevented any further outbreaks following the epidemic in the 1890s.

Dysentery could not be dealt with in the same simple manner. It remained intractable, and each newly opened district was affected by it. Sanitary measures were only slowly introduced. Clean water was brought to a few villages on the Gazelle Peninsula; no such improvements were made in other districts, with the exception of Manus, where the 1912 dysentery epidemic stirred the government into quick action. Venereal diseases were perceived early as a threat to the population, but compulsory medical examination and, if necessary, treatment of all labourers before taking up work on a plantation did not overcome the problem. Inevitably some infected labourers evaded examination or treatment was incomplete. But venereal infections prevailed also in the vicinity of European centres and doctors were unable to do anything other than treat each case as it came before them. Tuberculosis grew from a little noticed problem to one that was seen as a potentially serious threat to New Guineans, but there are no indications as to how the authorities proposed to prevent its spread.

At an individual level doctors carried out some useful work in villages. Potentially much more useful was their training of medical *tultuls*. By teaching some basic medical skills, villagers were empowered to deal with the most common afflictions. Whether the other objective was achieved—paving the way for easy access to villagers by doctors to treat diseases that doctors thought were important—was never fully tested as the travelling doctor scheme was introduced only just before the outbreak of war.

Weighed against the positive side are the detrimental effects of colonisation on the health of the population. Malaria became more widespread so that an increasing number of people became victims of its pernicious effects. With the exception of cholera and smallpox, newly introduced infectious diseases had a severe and long-term impact, one which lasted well beyond the German period.

The motivation for German interest in the health of the population was their dependence on New Guinean labour. Health was narrowly perceived by the authorities as physical fitness for plantation work and raising a large family. Medical care in villages had to embrace the whole family, men, women and children. Concerned with the effects of a declining population on the economy, the administration's attention could no longer centre only on the labour force, mostly men; all villagers had to be integrated into a medical system, but in particular it had to encompass women and children. This was the essential point of intervention to generate population growth, a guarantee that the colony would flourish.

CONCLUSION

Has it all been worthwhile?

Many a German doctor, being deported from New Guinea when war broke out, might have asked "Has it all been worthwhile?", as Professor Black did in 1966 when he reviewed achievements of western medicine in Papua and New Guinea.[1]

Some German doctors had spent many years in the colony. Dempwolff, who had come back early in 1914 for the third time and was deported on H.M.S. *Berrima* in November 1914, could look back on an association of nearly twenty years. He had first worked in Kaiser-Wilhelmsland when conditions were precarious; doctors knew little of how to deal with malaria, the cardinal threat to the health of all; mortality and morbidity were exceptionally high, and nursing facilities were primitive. Early in the century he had returned to work on malaria control, only to discover that, although malaria could be eradicated in theory, in practice it was a very complex task. When he came back in 1914—this time to pursue linguistic studies—he found that progress had been made in a decade.

The German administration had built up a medical service which was available to all people, Europeans and natives alike, living within the control of the government. Starting with one doctor in 1886, by 1914 eight were employed by the government.[2] Eleven medical orderlies were working for the govern-

---

1   Editorial, *PNGMedJ* 9(3) 1966: 77
2   1 Senior medical officer based in Rabaul, 2 medical officers in Rabaul, and 1 each in Herbertshöhe, Kaewieng, Namatanai, Kieta, Friedrich-Wilhelmshafen

ment, some with doctors in native hospitals, others as the only medical authority on a station.[3] A similar number of privately employed medical orderlies were working in plantation hospitals.[4] At the European hospitals Red Cross nurses were working,[5] and in villages *Heiltultuls* were dressing ulcers and dispensing cough mixtures and quinine.

Unlike the early days, new settlers from Germany could now expect good medical and nursing care in a pleasant and well managed hospital in the capital, and new hospitals were on the drawing board for Kaewieng and Friedrich-Wilhelmshafen. Housing for Europeans was built well separated from contact with the local population. New Guinea had become safe enough for men to bring their wives; and single men could be encouraged to marry German women and settle in the colony. With facilities at the hospital also tailored to the needs of women and children, there was every chance that they could raise a family, secure in the knowledge that medical and nursing care was available if need arose.

Doctors could take some credit for making the colonial venture possible for Germans in New Guinea. Although powerless and hard pressed to claim much success in the early years, when malaria control became possible they applied the new methods swiftly, and prescribed appropriate doses of quinine prophylactically and therapeutically. Even though not all expatriates strictly followed doctors' instructions on quinine prophylaxis, the majority of settlers could work in the tropics for years, unlike before the turn of the century, when many returned home because of ill health or died prematurely.

The government had also built hospitals for natives. Doctors spent a considerable amount of their time there and in plantation hospitals maintained by big firms. Their contribution to the maintenance of the labour force was important. They had treated innumerable labourers for tropical ulcers and probably nearly as many with other skin complaints. They tried to bring malaria under control and dispensed large quantities of quinine, equally large quantities of castor oil to treat dysentery, and uncounted mercury treatments for venereal disease. They had been unstinting in the use of expectorants to ease bronchial infections, and other medications to relieve pain and discomfort. Large quantities of disinfectants and antiseptics had killed off a lot of dangerous bacteria. Doctors had also found that balanced nutrition could

---

3   2 in Herbertshöhe, 2 in Rabaul, 1 in Kaewieng, 1 in Namatanai, 1 in Kieta, 1 in Friedrich-Wilhelmshafen; one medical orderly worked independently in each of Eitape, Morobe and Manus.

4   New Guinea Company at least 4, Forsayth & Co., Wahlen, and BAG all at least one.

5   2 in Rabaul, 1 in Herbertshöhe, and 1 in Friedrich-Wilhelmshafen.

cure easily and prevent beriberi, and they were attempting to educate employers to improve labourers' diet. They had advised the government that health would improve with sanitation, clean water, and attention to mosquito breeding grounds. Where improvements had been made, it had been at their behest.

Doctors had tried to find ways of encouraging villagers to make use of medical services and had not hesitated to use the latest drugs available from Germany. People suffered from many ills which medical treatment could cure or ameliorate. The long, slow process of gaining the confidence of the people was still going on. Gradually those living near European settlements were taking advantage of medical services and consulting a doctor for some complaints. A new drug had come onto the market with which the ubiquitous yaws could be successfully treated; doctors began to use it freely, and yaws-afflicted people consulted doctors; there was no need to impose treatment. Doctors had saved or prolonged lives by treating afflictions of the indigenous people, and many of these enjoyed a better quality of life because they were treated not for life-threatening conditions, but for complaints that were unpleasant or debilitating. Over the years many thousands had been protected against smallpox; vaccination was still going on in the Toma district when Australian troops arrived.

The converse of the strategy, bringing medicine to the people instead of waiting for them to come and ask for it, looked promising with the introduction of the *Heiltultul*. With newly acquired skills, some basic medications and dressings, *tultuls* were able to treat some of the most common disorders of villagers.

What was perhaps most frustrating for Dempwolff was the thought that, when doctors were at long last provided with more funds to carry out their work and bring health to the native population, their efforts were cut short by the outbreak of war. He and other doctors had written innumerable reports on native health and made dozens of recommendations on how to improve it. It had been a long battle by doctors; their efforts were thwarted for years by lack of resources. At the very moment when their goals were within reach—more funds for health services, and natives gaining confidence in western medicine—their endeavours came to nothing. At most he could hope that the Australians would continue where German doctors had been compelled to leave off.

We now leave Dempwolff to his ruminations, take a less doctor-centred perspective, and reflect on wider issues of public health.

From the beginning of German colonisation, medical services were closely related to colonial interests. When Germans first set up camp in Finschhafen in the mid-1880s, a doctor was sent to look after their health. It was known that malaria was endemic on the Kaiser-Wilhelmsland coast, but its virulence was not appreciated, nor its likely effect on colonists and the small labour force they brought to the country.

Morbidity and mortality among the newcomers were very high in the early years. Advances in medical science, allocation of considerable resources to a small number of people, combined with nutritional improvements, adequate sanitation and racial segregation, all played a part in ensuring better health so that a generation later New Guinea no longer presented the same dangers to colonists. Settling permanently and raising a family had become feasible. In the language of the time, Germans were becoming acclimatised in New Guinea.

For the labour force, brought in increasing numbers from south-east Asia and the Bismarck Archipelago to Kaiser-Wilhelmsland, health conditions were appalling for many years with exceedingly high mortality. A high labour mortality was typical in the early years of plantation development elsewhere but, because of high malaria endemicity, levels reached in German New Guinea up to the turn of the century were far in excess of other Pacific plantation economies at a similar stage of development. People, weakened by malaria and malnourished, readily fell prey to infectious diseases, rife in unsanitary conditions. But even when malaria control became possible, and large-scale importation of the highly vulnerable Asian coolies had ceased, frequent dysentery and beriberi epidemics suggested that a better diet and sanitation should be foremost to ensure better health. Such improvements depended on the political will and power of the government to compel employers to make necessary changes. An attempt in 1909 to improve labourers' rations fell short when the proposed Labour Ordinance came up against the determination of planters to keep their costs minimal. Unlike a traditional diet, polished rice was a cheap and convenient way of feeding large numbers of people. A regular supply of traditional foods throughout the year would have demanded labour and land—both more profitably used to grow copra. A renewed attempt in 1913 to improve conditions—with ration proposals based on a traditional diet and scientifically determined nutritional requirements—was still under discussion when war broke out.

However, the newcomers were not the only ones adversely affected. They themselves brought infectious diseases which spread to the local population.

Colonisation altered the epidemiological climate rapidly, and New Guineans were exposed to a number of infectious diseases against which they had no immunity. Recurrence of cholera was prevented with quarantine; vaccination and quarantine were also effective in preventing smallpox, but only after an outbreak claimed an unknown number of victims. Other infectious diseases were more insidious and not amenable to quarantine. Influenza reached New Guinea in the early 1890s, decimating a malaria-weakened labour force and also costing uncounted lives in villages. Venereal infections proved intractable. Little notice was taken at first of tuberculosis, at a time when doctors were overwhelmed with other health problems. Only after the turn of the century, when malaria came under some control, did doctors begin to look more closely at other disorders, and notice the growing number of tubercular infections, many resulting in death. Introduced by infected Europeans and repatriated labourers, the spread of tuberculosis was a growing health threat.

Gastro-enteric diseases were a chronic problem. Improvement depended on changes in personal habits, but colonisers displayed a curious attitude to change. They expected New Guineans to accept change, such as adopting different work habits and tools, or dealing with injury and disease by consulting a doctor, not to mention conversions sought by missionaries. Yet administrators and planters were reluctant to introduce new sanitary habits—which could not be effected unless there were good water supplies and latrines— on the grounds that people were unlikely to forego their old ways. Labourers were therefore not taught new methods of hygiene once they left their villages, and traditional ways of disposing of sanitary waste posed a serious health hazard in crowded conditions. When the government finally improved conditions for its work force in Rabaul, planters procrastinated; sanitary conditions remained dubious, and dysentery, with its high mortality rate, persisted on plantations.

The attitude of planters was very short-sighted: although they asserted frequently that a labour shortage hampered rapid plantation development, they did not make the best possible use of labourers available by ensuring their good health. Rational management surely dictated that sound nutrition, clean water and malaria prophylaxis were less costly than an average labour morbidity of around 8 per cent, and even higher during epidemics. It seems that early in the century, when mortality rates dropped, complacency set in. Planters accepted a certain level of morbidity and mortality and, compared with the early years in Kaiser–Wilhelmsland, the situation had undoubtedly improved. Appeals to planters' self-interest fell on deaf ears; another attempt to improve labour conditions was still being negotiated when war broke out.

Increased population movement through recruitment, and greater contact between villages under government control, had other unforeseen consequences: malaria was introduced into non-malarious districts, or new types of malaria were introduced where only one type was endemic. When effects became obvious, it was not a matter of changing the direction of colonial development, but of finding ways to ameliorate problems created by colonisation. Disease and ill health were never allowed to stand in the way of colonial advances. The hope that scientific research would find the way to eradicate malaria seemed fulfilled when the malaria cycle was discovered, and research by Professor Koch in New Guinea confirmed that effective intervention was possible. Koch's proposal for malaria eradication was to break the cycle in people by identifying with blood tests all parasite carriers, in particular non-clinical cases, and treating them with quinine. Based on the theory of identifying and destroying a pathogen, this method was successful in a small scale experiment in Bogadjim, but its large-scale application was a Herculean task. The cost of such a program in a country with a widely dispersed population in difficult terrain was beyond available resources and large scale malaria eradication was quietly dropped from health plans. Instead—with Europeans the most important group to be protected from malaria—segregation of races became the accepted policy, most clearly demonstrated in the planning of the capital, Rabaul. Attempts were made with ecological control, but systematic infilling of mosquito breeding grounds came up against the apathy of householders and planters and a shortage of funds, even though it proved effective in reducing the incidence of malaria wherever it was carried out.

When the Reich took over the administration, the relationship between medical services and economic interests became even stronger than during the New Guinea Company period, when attention turned to extending health control to villages where population numbers were seen to be falling. While the problem was described as population decline, it was labour shortage that motivated government intervention. The labour question dominated colonial politics, and the need for a large labour force determined health policies. The fundamental resource of the country was its population, and its survival and growth was crucial for the viability of the colony. Two courses of action were deemed appropriate to promote health and growth. One was to intervene in traditional practices—birth control and blood feuds—believed to prevent population growth. The other was to improve the health of villagers with western medical techniques.

Whether the population was in fact declining has to remain unanswered, with the exception of isolated islands and atolls where, following the introduction of malaria, sudden drops in small, self-contained populations were conspicuous. There is less certainty in other districts under German control. Early censuses were often estimates based on unreliable information, and not enough counts had been made to indicate clear demographic trends by 1914. However, a precariously balanced population in a malarial region was likely to suffer a check from recurrent epidemics of newly introduced infectious diseases.[6] That being the case, recurring dysentery epidemics from the early 1880s onwards and influenza epidemics in the early 1890s on the Gazelle Peninsula and in New Ireland probably had a negative impact on population numbers. The demographic effect of venereal diseases is an unknown factor. So is the impact of the introduction of other malaria types and the spread of malaria to non-malarious regions on the Gazelle Peninsula and in New Ireland. In Kaiser-Wilhelmsland dysentery was not as severe as in the Bismarck Archipelago, and its impact on population numbers is not known, nor is that of influenza epidemics in the early 1890s, which were followed by smallpox.

By 1914, when numerous population surveys had been made, reports by the Chief Medical Officer in particular suggest that there were several points of intervention. One was an improvement in water supplies; the few village wells installed on the Gazelle Peninsula and on Manus were barely a first step towards improving sanitary conditions in villages. The role of malaria and tuberculosis in public health was being reassessed; malaria had a continual effect and tuberculosis had potentially serious effects. Another critical point of intervention was in maternal and child care. Unless more children survived infancy and childhood, population numbers would at best remain static. Plans for large families for New Guineans were based on European needs and perceptions and little thought was given to likely effects of a sudden population growth on New Guineans. The health of women was of concern because it affected their capacity to bear children. Fundamental economic changes—the transformation of a subsistence economy to a plantation economy—necessarily had to be accompanied by fundamental social changes.

Doctors played an important role in shaping health policies and strategies

---

6   John Burton's study 'A Dysentery Epidemic in New Guinea and its Mortality' in *JPH* 18.3/4(1983): 236-61 shows the complexity of assessing the demographic impact of an epidemic.

over their thirty years in New Guinea. A gradual process can be observed by which they increased their influence, in keeping with a growing confidence in their ability to deal with health problems. During the New Guinea Company period there was friction between doctors and management as they tried to determine their respective spheres of control. Doctors were at a disadvantage; they were subordinate to company management, and also lacked confidence in their professional abilities as they were quite obviously unable to deal with the health problems they confronted. This changed rapidly at the turn of the century when, as government employees, they were no longer responsible to plantation managements. More importantly, their inability to deal with health problems brought to the fore a narrowly defined field of 'tropical medicine' in which doctors needed special knowledge. With the establishment of an institute for tropical diseases came specialist training, a boost to confidence and status; doctors became the acknowledged experts to deal with the colony's health problems.

Ironically, despite their specialist training in tropical medicine, the fundamental health policy doctors proposed to protect colonists was based on time-honoured quarantine, specifically the segregation of races. The creation of white enclaves on health grounds fostered a notion that whites would be healthy but for contact with malaria-infected and untreatable blacks. A later discovery that white children were infected with hookworm reinforced the perception that racial segregation was essential for the safety of Europeans. Earlier views that New Guinea and its climate were responsible for ill-health were modified: the problem was not with the country, but with its people, and ostensibly there were valid grounds to ensure that Namanula, the suburb on the slopes above Rabaul, would remain a white domain, and to encourage settlers to build their residences well away from labourers' barracks. The correlation of disease with race was not new; it was common before the turn of the century when explanations for high labour mortality were sought, but it did not at that time lead to racial segregation. However, the earlier correlation was based on the belief that physiological differences between races accounted for particular diseases. Bacteriological research established that 'germs' were the cause of disease, irrespective of the colour of the people. Racial segregation was therefore the means to create a healthy environment for Europeans, but also a tacit admission of failure in dealing with public health.

Doctors also determined that medical services would be hospital-based, and by 1914 all districts under German control either had European and native hospitals, or plans for their construction were well advanced. Hospitals had to be set up to accommodate the sick, the majority of whom were without families or other support. Hospitals, and out-patients departments that usually went with them, were the responsibility of doctors. There they exerted control directly, or indirectly through the nursing staff.

Doctors only ever had limited influence in determining health aspects of labour policies. Planters strongly opposed interference in the management of their labour force and the doctor's role was that of therapist.

Policies and strategies for medical services for villages were the most important sphere, potentially affecting the whole population under German control. For about a decade a lack of resources, together with a reluctance of villagers to make use of what medical services there were, meant that a limited number of individuals were treated for specific disorders, but there were no mass campaigns apart from smallpox vaccination. However, doctors tried to gain increasing autonomy in village health programs, as is evident from the writings by the newly appointed Chief Medical Officer who envied the greater power and independence of doctors in British colonies and called for the appointment of doctors as district officers. Underlying this was a quest for more independence and greater influence by the medical profession in formulating and implementing public health policies, as well as for more resources. A dual role of administrator and doctor would give great scope for monitoring villages and implementing health programs.[7]

However, before doctors could do much work in villages, ways had to be found to persuade villagers to make use of the medical services offered and adopt western medical techniques to deal with illness. Of the two proposals, that for *Heiltultuls* was implemented immediately, probably as much for its small cost as for its potential for paving the way for doctors, or for teaching New Guineans new skills. Before the second proposal, the appointment of travelling doctors, could be implemented, new German drugs gave doctors a chance to demonstrate the superiority of their medicine. Arsphenamines cured the ubiquitous yaws swiftly and effectively and, as villagers began to seek medical help for this complaint on seeing the efficacy of the treatment, raised doctors' hopes that villagers would consult them also for other disorders.

Policy proposals for health programs fell into two periods: the first from the time the Reich assumed power to around 1912, the second for the two years to the end of German rule. Policy decisions in the first period were reflected in the 1914 budget, when the scene was set for an extension of medical services

---

7   Külz, 'Grundzüge der kolonialen Eingeborenenhygiene', 5

to villages and hamlets, with yaws and hookworm the foci of attention of mass campaigns. This approach, later also taken by Australian doctors, confirms a view that "new therapeutic possibilities often persuaded medical authorities to devote their attention and resources to previously tolerated suffering."[8] Yaws, although very common in New Guinea, was rarely a life-threatening disorder, and before the advent of arsphenamines, only the most unsightly cases were treated, and not always successfully. Yet, by 1914 yaws featured large as a serious disease in need of eradication. Hookworm was targeted because it caused debilitating anaemia. However, although malaria was more debilitating, its eradication had been abandoned because there was no cheap, effective and simple method. But hookworm therapy was available, and was suitable to be used in a mass health campaign. Targeting a specific disease was typical of the narrow discipline of tropical medicine which, in its bacteriological method, largely neglected wider health problems. This resulted in the ironic situation that New Guineans were to enjoy the blessings of arsphenamines—the newest drugs produced by German pharmacology—before they had water wells. Hookworm eradication meant treatment of the population, but not sanitary measures, so that hookworm infestation remained in the ground and readily reinfected the population.

However, although the 1914 budget for village programs was narrowly based on perceptions of tropical medicine, I suggest that a turning point had been reached and, under the direction of the Chief Medical Officer, a broader approach was to be taken. With his slogan "Latrines and clean water!"[9] he argued for raising standards of village hygiene. He had been urging for years that hygienic measures were as essential as any mass health campaign, and that the health of mothers and children was a priority in creating a healthy and plentiful population. His prescription was for much wider measures than those encompassed by tropical medicine. He assessed health problems in New Guinea by comparing them to backward rural regions in Germany some decades earlier and proposed measures similar to those that had been effective there in bringing about general improvements. Health programs, such as mother and infant care, which were put into effect in contemporary Germany, were also appropriate in New Guinea.

Implementation of policies depended in the last instance on resources.

8   Donald Denoon, *Public health in Papua New Guinea: Medical possibility and social constraint, 1884-1984* (Cambridge: Cambridge University Press, 1989) 2
9   Külz, 'Die seuchenhaften Krankheiten des Kindesalters der Eingeborenen und ihre Bedeutung für die koloniale Bevölkerungsfrage', *Koloniale Rundschau* 1913: 329

Pressure from New Guinea alone for more health funds was not enough; a change of attitudes in Berlin was as important. In the last years before the war, opinions on native policies were reshaped in Berlin by different pressure groups. In colonial circles the view that population decline had to be reversed was gaining acceptance. A eugenic movement was advancing counter-measures to combat an apparent population decline in Germany, and favourably influenced colonial debates. The allocation of more funds for medical services in German New Guinea in 1913[10] and 1914, together with a grant for two travelling doctors reflected a new attitude to colonial health.

Germans probably came closest to meeting immediate needs of New Guineans with the introduction of the *Heiltultul* system. The basic skills a *tultul* learnt enabled him to attend the most common afflictions of villagers. It was a transfer of skills which empowered villagers to deal with health problems. Whether the ulterior motive for training *tultuls* was achieved—to encourage villagers to consult a doctor—is uncertain; the system operated for too short a period to judge its long term impact. In implementing the program, doctors came up against an unexpected complication: they could not impose a *tultul* on a village without villagers' approval, but they remained silent on how they handled village politics.

Plans for medical research in New Guinea foundered early. It is doubtful that this was any loss to the people of New Guinea. First-class research was being carried out in Germany, for instance at the Institute for Infectious Diseases in Berlin, and the Institute for Ships' and Tropical Medicine in Hamburg. An improvement in living standards for New Guineans depended not so much on high technology achievements, as on low technology measures, such as good water supplies, or new ways of disposing of waste and sewage hygienically, a condition of which the newly appointed Chief Medical Officer was well aware.

There was in any case a dichotomy between scientific research on tropical diseases in Germany and activities in the colony. Malaria serves as an example: while scientists gained more and more insights into the etiology of malaria and the morphology and development of malaria parasites, in New Guinea the infection was spread into non-malarious regions, and recruits from the Bismarck Archipelago were exposed to new varieties of malaria on arrival in Kaiser-Wilhelmsland which they carried with them on repatriation. Laboratory research in Germany did nothing to prevent this new health threat. Field research, on the other hand, brought awkward and unwelcome

10   The extra allocation in 1913 was for medical services in the Island Territory.

results, as was the case with Dempwolff's field work in New Guinea. The main conclusion was that malaria was spreading because of colonial activities, but a mass malaria eradication campaign was beset with enormous difficulties and costs. It was safer to settle for research in a laboratory.

New Guineans were never consulted when doctors decided what was important and what was not in the interests of New Guineans. Their voice could be heard every so often in their reluctance to consult a doctor, in their absconding from hospital, but also in their decision to seek a doctor's help where he obviously and miraculously could help.

Doctors and administrators had spent nearly three decades attempting to come to grips with health problems in New Guinea when the German colonial experiment came to an abrupt end. It was at a time when new far-reaching policies were in the offing. We can only speculate on the speed with which they would have been implemented and the resources allocated for them. The pity is that Australian doctors paid little attention to the point which their predecessors had reached, and did not go on in the direction that was signposted but, as Donald Denoon has clearly and concisely shown in his *Public Health in Papua New Guinea*, started their own colonial experiments.

GESUNDHEITSWESEN UND KOLONIALISMUS
DER FALL DEUTSCH-NEUGUINEA
1884-1914

KOLONISATION UND ÄRZTE

Die Grundlagen des kolonialen Gesundheitswesens wurden durch den Wissensstand der Zeit und die damit zusammenhängende Einstellung der Ärzte bestimmt. Infolge des raschen Fortschritts in der wissenschaftlichen Forschung in den 1870er und 1880er Jahren und dank der Entdeckung von Aseptik, Antiseptik, besonderen Bakterien als Krankheitserregern und neuen Diagnosemethoden, wuchs das Ansehen der Ärzte und damit ihr Einfluß und ihre Macht. Tropenmedizin wurde zu einer völlig neuen Spezialwissenschaft, die die allgemeine Richtung des Gesundheitswesens in den Kolonien elementar beeinflußte. Eine große Rolle spielten nicht zuletzt rassenhygienische Theorien, die auch in Deutsch-Neuguinea ein Echo fanden.

Es muß betont werden, daß die Entwicklungen auf wissenschaftlichem und sozialtheoretischem Gebiet und die sich herausbildende Tropenmedizin sich nicht auf Deutschland beschränkten. Ganz ähnliche Vorgänge und Verhaltensmuster lassen sich bei anderen Kolonialmächten in dieser Zeit nachweisen.

Als Neuguinea 1884 annektiert wurde, war allgemein akzeptiert, daß das Klima die Gesundheit des Menschen in direkter und indirekter Weise beeinflußte. Die Frage, wie sich Deutsche in den neuen Kolonien akklimatisieren könnten, wurde zuerst von Rudolf Virchow aufgeworfen. Virchow hegte schwere Bedenken gegen die Ansiedlung von Weißen in tropischen Malariagebieten. Andererseits war er jedoch überzeugt, daß die medizinische Forschung die kolonialen Gesundheitsprobleme lösen würde. Virchow vertrat die Ansicht, daß Krankheitsursachen und Epidemien durch ein komplexes Ineinandergreifen von pathologischen Ursachen, sozialen Bedingungen, wirtschaftlichen Interessen und politischem Gestalten erklärt werden konnten. Weder einfache Lösungen noch zentral gesteuerte Maßnahmen würden eine Verbesserung der öffentlichen Gesundheit herbeiführen, sondern es mußten die lokalen Gegebenheiten, d.h. die konkreten sozialen, wirtschaftlichen und politischen Umstände vor Ort, in die Planung mit einbezogen werden. Der Einfluß des in der wissenschaftlichen Medizin führenden Professor Robert Koch auf die Entwicklung der Tropenmedizin war jedoch für die allgemeine Richtung des kolonialen Gesundheitswesens lange maßgebend. Kochs Theorien im Kampf gegen Krankheiten beruhten auf der Erkennung des Krankheitserregers, seiner Isolierung und seiner schließlichen Zerstörung.

Die Tropenmedizin war eine jener medizinischen Fachwissenschaften, die gegen Ende des 19. Jahrhunderts entstanden. Ursprünglich bezog sich der Ausdruck "Tropenhygiene" ausschließlich auf die Gesundheit der in den Tropen wohnenden Europäer. Später wurde er auch auf die Gesundheit aller Tropenbewohner bezogen. Der Ausdruck "tropische Krankheit" und "tropische Medizin" wurde erst allmählich verwendet, möglicherweise unter dem Einfluß eines Artikels, der im Jahre 1898 im *Journal of Tropical Medicine* erstmals erschien.

In den 1880er und Anfang der 90er Jahre beruhte die tropenhygienische Forschung auf der Sammlung von statistischem Material über die spezifischen lokalen Bedingungen wie Wetter, Krankheitsarten, Krankheitsvorkommen und Mortalität, sowie auf dem Vergleich der Physiologie der verschiedenen Menschenrassen. Unterstützt von der Kolonialgesellschaft sandte der "Verein Deutscher Naturforscher und Ärzte" 1891 und 1894 einen Fragebogen an Ärzte in tropischen Ländern und Kolonien. Die Resultate waren unbefriedigend. Es zeigte sich, daß eine Einrichtung wissenschaftlicher Labors in den Kolonien nötig war, und ein entsprechender Vorschlag wurde dem Reichstag unterbreitet. Nach langwierigen Verhandlungen wurde mit einem Zuschuß des Kolonialamts und der Stadt im Jahre 1900 in Hamburg das Institut für Schiffs- und Tropenhygiene gegründet.

Die Aufgabe dieses Instituts war die Ausbildung der Ärzte zur Erforschung und Diagnostizierung tropischer Krankheiten. Von 1897 an wurde die Zeitschrift *Archiv für Schiffs- und Tropenhygiene* regelmäßig herausgegeben und trug so zur Verbreitung des neuen Wissensstandes unter Ärzten und Forschern bei.

Im Jahre 1907 wurde die deutsche tropenmedizinische Gesellschaft gegründet. Die Öffentlichkeit wurde mit dem Begriff der Tropenmedizin durch Ausstellungen, wie z.B. die internationale Hygieneausstellung in Dresden 1911, bekannt gemacht.

Die sogenannte Rassenhygiene, ein Begriff, der sich aus Theorien des Sozialdarwinismus entwickelte, fand auch den Weg in die koloniale Gesundheitspolitik. Um die Jahrhundertwende, als sich vorwiegend in Industriestädten eine deutliche Geburtenabnahme zeigte, wurde dieser Bevölkerungsrückgang als eine Bedrohung der politischen Stärke Deutschlands und ein Zeichen von Degeneration betrachtet. Eine Debatte über den Bevölkerungsrückgang fand auch in den Kolonien statt, wo man glaubte, ähnliche Zustände beobachten zu können. Entvölkerung oder eine Eingeborenenbevölkerung, die krankheitshalber nicht in der Lage war, zu arbeiten, galten als ebenso schwere Bedrohung der Plantagenkolonien wie die Malaria.

Gleich zu Beginn der deutschen Kolonisation wurden in den Kolonien Ärzte zur Gesundheitsversorgung eingestellt. In Deutsch-Neuguinea waren die Ärzte anfänglich nicht durchgehend mit medizinischen Aufgaben beschäftigt. Die Zahl der Patienten war klein und die Behandlungsmöglichkeiten eingeschränkt, da eine effiziente Behandlung des größten Problems, der Malaria, noch nicht bekannt war. Viele Ärzte unternahmen deshalb auch ethnographische Forschungen. Mit dem Anwachsen der Zahl von Plantagenarbeitern vergrößerte sich aber auch die Arbeit für die Ärzte. Die Behandlung von Malaria, Dysenterie, Beriberi und eitrigen Geschwüren gehörte zur täglichen Routine des Arztes. Nach der Jahrhundertwende zeichneten sich gewisse Änderungen ab. Theoretisch sollten die Ärzte jetzt einem, alle Kolonien umfassenden, Malaria-Forschungsteam angehören. In der Praxis war dieses Ziel in Deutsch-Neuguinea nicht erreichbar und die Ärzte beschränkten sich auf klinische Beobachtungen und ausführliche Berichte, die nach Berlin geschickt wurden. Krankenhäuser wurden jedoch besser ausgerüstet und man konnte mehr chirurgische Eingriffe vornehmen als vor 1900.

Die Verständigung zwischen den Ärzten und den eingeborenen Patienten war oft schwierig. Man mußte sich auf eine gemeinsame Sprache verständigen, was in den ersten Jahren auf Pidgin-Englisch hinauslief. Oft waren die Ärzte in ihren Diagnosen und ihrer Therapie unsicher.

Zur Zeit der Neuguinea-Compagnie wurden Ärzte von dieser Kompanie engagiert und bezahlt. Nachdem das Reich die Kolonie übernommen hatte, wurden Ärzte als Staatsangestellte eingestellt. Der erste staatlich angestellte Arzt war Dr. Wilhelm Wendland, der im November 1901 seine Arbeit in

Herbertshöhe auf der Gazellenhalbinsel aufnahm. Dr. Hoffmann, der erste Staatsarzt in Friedrich-Wilhelmshafen, fing dort im August 1902 an. Während der deutschen Kolonialzeit war immer nur ein Regierungsarzt in Kaiser-Wilhelmsland angestellt. Im Bismarck-Archipel vermehrte sich dagegen die Zahl der Ärzte: 1904 wurde in Käwieng eine Arztstelle eingerichtet, 1905 wurde ein zweiter Arzt für das Gebiet von Rabaul eingestellt, 1911 wurde ein Arzt in Namatanai (Neumecklenburg) eingesetzt und 1913 einer in Kieta auf den nördlichen Salomonen. Schließlich wurde im Jahre 1913 das Gesundheitswesen neu organisiert und eine Oberarztstelle für die ganze Kolonie, einschließlich des Inselgebietes (Mikronesien), geschaffen.

Zu den Zeiten der Neuguinea-Compagnie waren Spannungen zwischen der Kompanie und den Ärzten nahezu unvermeidlich. Auf der einen Seite verlangten die Ärzte volle Autorität in allen, das Gesundheitswesen betreffenden Angelegenheiten, auf der anderen Seite insistierte die Firma auf der strengen Beachtung ihrer wirtschaftlichen Interessen. Unannehmlichkeiten und Streitereien trugen neben den eigenen Krankheiten dazu bei, daß viele Ärzte ihren Vertrag mit der Firma nicht voll erfüllten und das Land vorzeitig verließen. Nur drei der fünfzehn von der Neuguinea-Compagnie angestellten Ärzte hielten ihren zwei- oder dreijährigen Vertrag auch voll ein.

Konflikte zwischen den Ärzten und der Regierung waren jedoch nicht allein auf die Verwaltungszeit der Neuguinea-Compagnie beschränkt, wie die Debatte um die neuzugründende Hauptstadt der Kolonie zeigt. Wirtschaftliche und militärpolitische Bedingungen hatten letzten Endes den ausschlaggebenden Einfluß, nicht die von den Ärzten geforderten gesundheitlichen Voraussetzungen.

Pläne für eine Malariaforschung durch staatlich angestellte Ärzte wurden in Deutsch-Neuguinea nie realisiert; die täglichen Schwierigkeiten, denen sich die Ärzte gegenüber sahen, füllten ihre gesamte Zeit aus. Nach der Jahrhundertwende konnten sie durch Chinin-Prophylaxe relativ malariafrei leben. Die allgemeinen Wohnungs- und Lebensbedingungen verbesserten sich ebenfalls langsam, und die Aussichten für eine längere Karriere als Arzt in Deutsch-Neuguinea wurden besser.

DER TROPENKRANKE EUROPÄER

Eine Unterschätzung der gesundheitlichen Gefahren und eine Nicht-beachtung der Warnung vor einer gesundheitsschädlichen Kolonisationspolitik hatten schwerwiegende Folgen für viele der Kolonialbewohner. Malaria war und blieb, trotz der von Robert Koch erweckten Hoffnung, das fortwährende und sich nur langsam verbessernde Gesundheitsproblem der Auswanderer. Theoretisch konnte Malaria zwar durch Chinin-Prophylaxe oder durch eine Chinin-Therapie überwunden werden. In der Praxis wurde die regelmäßige Chinin-Einnahme mit ihren unangenehmen Nebenerscheinungen jedoch nicht allgemein akzeptiert und eine obligatorische Chinin-Einnahme ließ sich nicht durchsetzen. Technische Maßnahmen, z.B. die Trockenlegung und Sauberhaltung der Umgebung zur Verminderung von Moskito-Brutstätten sowie eine Vergitterung von Türen und Fenstern, waren von öffentlicher Unterstützung und persönlicher Initiative abhängig und machten insgesamt nur langsam Fortschritte. Ein Erziehungsprogramm scheiterte nicht zuletzt auch an der Gleichgültigkeit und Nachlässigkeit der Menschen. Die Malariasituation im Kaiser-Wilhelmsland blieb prekär. Dort waren ungefähr 58% aller europäischen Todesfälle die direkte Folge von Malaria oder Schwarzwasserfieber, verglichen mit rund 22% im Bismarck-Archipel. Im letzteren war die Malariagefahr deutlich geringer und ganz generell zog man dort einen leichten Malariaanfall einer regelmäßigen prophylaktischen Chinin-Einnahme vor. Von 1902 an mußten sich alle Staatsangestellten einer ärztlichen Untersuchung für Tropendiensttauglichkeit unterziehen. Auf Siedler, Angestellte der Plantagengesellschaften und Missionare traf diese Vorschrift jedoch nicht zu. Die Gesundheit labiler Neuankömmlinge verschlimmerte sich daher rasch unter dem Einfluß von Malaria. Und auch von den Siedlern eingeschleppte Krankheiten gaben guten Grund zur Besorgnis. Tuberkulose, anfänglich kaum beachtet, galt 1914 für die einheimische Bevölkerung, die dagegen nicht immun war, als eine schwere Gefahr. Geschlechtskrankheiten, von Europäern und Chinesen eingeführt, erwiesen sich als hartnäckig und ihre Häufigkeit nahm trotz Maßnahmen und Vorschriften ständig zu.

Daß Selbsthilfe unerläßlich war, wurde als selbstverständlich akzeptiert, denn manche Ansiedler wohnten zu weit entfernt, um sofortige ärztliche Hilfe oder Medikamente zu erhalten. Besondere Bestimmungen für Apotheker in den Kolonien sollten eine Zufuhr von dubiosen Medikamenten aus fragwürdigen Quellen verhindern. Eine entsprechende, für alle Kolonien geltende Gesetzgebung, wurde aber erst am 1. Mai 1911 in Kraft gesetzt.

Von Anfang an ließ die Ernährungsbeschaffung einiges zu wünschen übrig. Lebensmittel mußten eingeführt werden, und da die Belieferung nicht zuverlässig war, gab es Engpässe. Aber auch als sich die Schiffsverbindungen verbesserten, blieb die Ernährungssituation der europäischen Bevölkerung nach ärztlicher Ansicht unbefriedigend, da zu wenig Frischwaren konsumiert wurden.

Krankenhausbauten zur Pflege der vielen Kranken erwiesen sich sehr bald als Notwendigkeit. Meistens waren die Neuankömmlinge unverheiratete europäische Männer, die im Krankheitsfall unversorgt waren, weil ihnen die häusliche Pflege einer Frau fehlte. Nach der Jahrhundertwende wurde die Notwendigkeit, Krankenhäuser zu bauen damit begründet, daß nunmehr europäische Frauen und Kinder in der Kolonie lebten und für deren Pflege ein Krankenhaus nötig sei. Gerade der erhoffte und erwartete Nachzug der Familien aus Deutschland war ein wichtiges Argument für den Ausbau der Gesundheitsfürsorge in den Kolonien.

Das notwendige Pflegepersonal in den Krankenhäusern für Europäer rekrutierte sich aus Pflegeschwestern, die zusammen mit einheimischen Helfern die eigentliche Krankenhausarbeit leisteten. Die Erhaltung eines Krankenhauses war im Verhältnis zur Anzahl der Patienten sehr teuer. Es waren jedoch Kosten, die zur Besserung der Gesundheitsverhältnisse der Ansiedler als unvermeidlich betrachtet wurden.

DIE ARBEITER

Die Plantagenunternehmen in Kaiser-Wilhelmsland waren ohne Rücksicht auf die Gesundheit der Arbeiterschaft gegründet worden. Zunächst wurden die Arbeiter aus Südostasien und aus dem Bismarck-Archipel importiert. Der Kontakt mit den in Neuguinea endemischen Krankheiten wirkte auf die ins Land gebrachten Arbeiter verhängnisvoll. Eine durch Infektionskrankheiten und unhygienische Lebensverhältnisse hervorgerufene hohe Mortalität war kennzeichnend für die Anfangsstadien aller Plantagenkolonien im pazifischen Raum, wobei Neuguinea die statistisch höchsten Mortalitätszahlen erreichte. Eine Besserung der Situation setzte nach ungefähr 15 Jahren ein und in Deutsch-Neuguinea war diese Verbesserung besonders markant.

Ärzte, die engagiert wurden, um die Gesundheit der Arbeitskräfte zu überwachen, waren in den ersten Jahren gegenüber den vorherrschenden Krankheiten nahezu machtlos. Da sie wenig zur Heilung beitragen konnten, versuchten sie, die prekären Gesundheitsverhältnisse zu erforschen. Solche Nachforschungen kamen immer auf den gleichen Punkt zurück: den Zusammenhang zwischen dem Klima und dem allgemeinen Gesundheitszustand, d.h. der Anpassungsfähigkeit der Neuankömmlinge. Der angeblich auf rassische Unterschiede zurückzuführende allgemeine schlechte Gesundheitszustand der Arbeiter war nach Meinung der Ärzte ein weiterer Grund der hohen Mortalität. Zwei fundamentale Probleme wurden nicht richtig erkannt: Erstens wurden die Arbeiter von einem epidemiologischen Klima in ein anderes versetzt, wo sie neuen Krankheiten ausgesetzt waren, gegen die sie nicht immun waren, gleichzeitig schleppten sie selbst Infektionskrankheiten in ihre neue Umgebung ein. Zweitens wurde durch die künstliche Zusammenballung großer Menschenmassen ohne die entsprechenden sanitären Einrichtungen höchst unhygienische Verhältnisse geschaffen.

Gesetzliche Vorschriften waren in ihrer Wirkung eingeschränkt wenn sie, wie die Einführung der Pocken zeigte, nicht genau befolgt wurden. Quarantänevorschriften wurden nach dem Ausbruch der Pockenepidemie in 1893 stärker befolgt und Impfungen für Arbeiter obligatorisch gemacht.

Nach der Jahrhundertwende verbesserten sich die Gesundheitsverhältnisse der Arbeiter. Die von Koch vorgeschriebene Behandlung brachte eine relative Verbesserung der Malariasituation auch unter der Arbeiterschaft, obwohl Malaria nicht ausrottbar war.

Ruhr war und blieb ein hartnäckiges Problem—ein Zeichen, daß die hygienischen Zustände gehoben werden mußten. Sanitäre Einrichtungen, einschließlich einer Wasserversorgung, wurden in die Planung der neuen Hauptstadt Rabaul einbezogen und die dortigen Verhältnisse gestalteten sich durch diese Neuerungen rasch günstiger. Auf Plantagen blieb jedoch alles beim alten. Ruhrepidemien wiederholten sich regelmäßig. Eine Änderung der unhygienischen Bedingungen auf den Plantagen wurde nur teilweise und langsam unternommen, so daß im Jahre 1914 noch immer ein Drittel aller Todesfälle auf Plantagen der Ruhr zugeschrieben wurden. Auf abgelegenen Plantagen, wo die Verhältnisse nur selten kontrolliert werden konnten, blieb die Lage prekär.

Die Ernährung der Arbeiter trug ebenfalls zur Krankheitsinzidenz bei. Mit wachsender Arbeiterzahl wurde es für die Plantagenbesitzer am billigsten und einfachsten, Reis als Hauptnahrungsmittel zu verabreichen. Diese einseitige Ernährung führte rasch zu Ausbrüchen von Beriberi, einer Vitaminmangelkrankheit, die auch in anderen europäischen Plantagenkolonien ein besonderes Problem darstellte. Die aus dem niederländischen Forschungsinstitut in Batavia kommende Nachricht über ausgezeichnete Erfolge mit Diätmodifikation—der Zugabe von "Katjang idjoe—Bohnen" (*phaseolus aureus*)— erreichte auch Deutsch-Neuguinea. Ähnliche Versuche mit Beriberi-Patienten ergaben so gute Ergebnisse, daß eine von der Regierung unterstützte "Bohnenkampagne" unternommen wurde. Die Wissenschaft hatte damit eine Antwort auf eine Krankheit gefunden, die die direkte Folge der Kolonisation war. Die nächste Aufgabe war nun, Plantagenbesitzer zu überzeugen, daß eine Verpflegung, die der traditionellen Kost der Arbeiter entsprach, für alle Seiten vorteilhafter wäre.

Die richtige Verpflegung der Arbeiter verursachte jahrelange Auseinandersetzungen zwischen der Regierung und den Plantagenunternehmern. Fortschritte in der wissenschaftlichen Forschung hoben die Wichtigkeit einer richtigen Ernährung hervor. In diesem Zusammenhang brachten die Ärzte die unbefriedigenden Gesundheitsverhältnisse mehr und mehr mit der ungeeigneten Nahrung in Verbindung. Die staatliche Festlegung von Verpflegungsvorschriften wurde jedoch von Plantageneigentümern als eine Bevorzugung der Arbeiter bewertet. Obwohl sich die Pflanzer ständig über Arbeitermangel beklagten, nutzten sie die vorhandene Arbeitskraft nicht richtig, da sie nicht alles taten, was möglich war, um die Arbeiterschaft bei guter Gesundheit zu erhalten.

Von Anfang an wurden auf den Plantagen schlichte Krankenhäuser zu Pflege der kranken Arbeiter gebaut. Bei Kriegsausbruch 1914 gab es außer den Plantagenkrankenhäusern der Firmen auch gut eingerichtete, von der Regierung erbaute Krankenhäuser für alle Eingeborenen. In diesen waren deutsche Krankenpfleger für den jeweiligen Spitalhaushalt und den Ablauf der täglichen Arbeit verantwortlich. Obschon der Bau und Unterhalt dieser Krankenhäuser im Verhältnis zur Bettenbesetzung nicht so teuer war wie der der Europäer-Krankenhäuser, verschlangen sie doch einen beträchtlichen Teil der Finanzen der kolonialen Gesundheitsbehörde. Die Notwendigkeit und Nützlichkeit der Krankenhäuser ist jedenfalls nicht bestreitbar. Es ist jedoch fraglich, ob ein Teil dieses Kostenaufwandes nicht besser zur Prävention von Krankheiten ausgegeben worden wäre.

DIE EINHEIMISCHE BEVÖLKERUNG

Der Zusammenhang zwischen Gesundheitswesen und wirtschaftlichen Interessen wurde enger, als das Reich 1899 die Verwaltung der Kolonie übernahm. Die Grundlage der wirtschaftlichen Entwicklung der Kolonie war die Eingeborenen-Bevölkerung, die in stets zunehmender Zahl als Plantagenarbeiter, aber auch in Bau- und Transportbetrieben eingesetzt wurde. Die Einführung von Arbeitskräften aus Südostasien hatte sich als erfolglos erwiesen, und die europäischen Siedler waren von Arbeitskräften innerhalb der Kolonie abhängig. Um den wachsenden Bedarf an Arbeitskräften sicherzustellen, war eine Zunahme der Eingeborenen-Bevölkerung erforderlich. Diese Prämisse setzte sich zu einer Zeit durch, als allgemein angenommen wurde, daß deren Zahlen sich verminderten oder, in extremen Fällen, ganze Stämme am aussterben waren. Eine gesunde Eingeborenen-Bevölkerung und die Entwicklung einer diesem Ziel gewidmeten Eingeborenen-Politik wurden deswegen zu vordringlichsten Aufgaben der Regierung.

Zunächst wurden Volkszählungen durchgeführt, um den Stand der Bevölkerung genau zu ermitteln. Diese Zählungen erwiesen sich aber als unzuverlässig, so daß ein wirklich allgemeingültiger demographischer Trend während der deutschen Kolonisation nicht klar festgestellt werden konnte. Zwei Maßnahmen wurden jedoch als nötig erachtet, um den angeblichen Bevölkerungsrückgang zu stoppen: Erstens mußte der Bevölkerung unter Mithilfe der Mission beigebracht werden, gewisse Verhaltensweisen zu ändern und zweitens mußte ein Sanitätsdienst zur Behandlung der Gesundheitsschäden in der Bevölkerung eingeführt werden. Und es war offensichtlich, daß staatlicherseits finanzielle Mittel zur Erreichung dieses Ziels zur Verfügung gestellt werden mußten.

Als Robert Koch Ende 1899 in Bogadjim mit Blutuntersuchungen und Chinin-Therapie ermutigende Ergebnisse erreichte, glaubte man, daß eine allgemeine Ausrottung der Malaria möglich wäre. Dr. Otto Dempwolff wurde nach Deutsch-Neuguinea gesandt, um Kochs Experimente zu wiederholen und anzuwenden. Dempwolff fand, daß Koch zu optimistisch gewesen war; die Topographie des Landes mit seinen weit voneinander entfernten Dörfern und Weilern präsentierte mannigfaltige Schwierigkeiten. Von großer Wichtigkeit war jedoch die Entdeckung, daß die Malaria auch in bisher malariafreie Gebiete vorgedrungen war, und daß neue Malariatypen in Gebieten mit bislang nur einem Malariatypus eingeführt worden waren. Bei dieser Verbreitung der Malaria spielte die Kolonisation ohne Frage eine führende Rolle. Durch Befriedung und Missionierung verstärkte und vervielfachte sich der Verkehr zwischen den zuvor eng voneinander abgegrenzten Dörfern und dadurch breitete sich die Malaria auch in zuvor nicht immunen Bevölkerungsgruppen aus. So brachten z.B. die von Kaiser-Wilhelmsland und dem Bismarck-Archipel zurückkehrenden Arbeiter einen neuen Malariatyp in ihre Heimatdörfer, der sich dann auch von dort aus verbreitete. Da es nicht möglich war, die Dorfbevölkerung von Malaria zu befreien, hieß es den Kontakt zwischen Eingeborenen und Europäern zur Verhütung ständiger Neuinfektionen zu vermeiden. Dies führte zu einer

Politik der Rassentrennung, die zum Beispiel in die Pläne für die neue Hauptstadt Rabaul mit einbezogen wurden. Die Verbindung Krankheit—Rasse war nicht neu und wurde oft als eine Erklärung für die hohe Arbeitermortalität gegeben. Eine solche Annahme basierte jedoch auf dem Axiom, daß physiologische Differenzen zwischen Rassen für unterschiedliche Krankheiten verantwortlich waren. Resultate der bakteriologischen Forschung ergaben, daß es pathogene Mikroorganismen waren, die Krankheiten verursachten und daß die Rasse dabei keine Rolle spielte. Rassentrennung war also weniger ein Mittel, die Gesundheit der Europäer abzusichern, sondern viel mehr ein Zugeständnis an die Unzulänglichkeiten des öffentlichen Gesundheitswesens. Auch die Ruhr wurde von den Plantagen in die Dörfer eingeschleppt, und die traditionelle Lebensweise der Melanesier führte zu einer raschen Ausbreitung der Infektion und zum regelmäßigen Aufflackern von Epidemien. In Rabaul und Umgebung verbesserte sich die Lage langsam mit dem Bau einer hygienischen Wasserversorgung für die Arbeiterviertel und die benachbarten Dörfer.

Die Integration der Eingeborenen in einen europäischen Gesundheitsdienst stieß auf Schwierigkeiten. Die einheimische Bevölkerung lebte in weit verstreuten Dörfern, der Gesundheitsdienst war dagegen in den kolonialen Siedlungen zentralisiert. Ein Weg mußte gefunden werden, um den Gesundheitsdienst in die Dörfer zu bringen. Eine Lösung war die Entwicklung des Heiltultul-Systems. Junge Männer wurden in einfachen Gesundheitsmaßnahmen ausgebildet und danach, ausgerüstet mit einigen Medikamenten und Verbandsmaterial, in ihre Dörfer zurückgeschickt. Dort verbanden sie Wunden, behandelten Geschwüre und oberflächliche Hautkrankheiten, verabreichten bei Fieber Chinin, bei Erkältung Hustenmittel. Bei Dysenterie isolierten sie die Patienten, verabreichten ihnen Rizinusöl und benutzten viel Desinfektionsmittel. Das Heiltultul-System hatte eine zweite, ebenso wichtige Funktion: Die Dorfbewohner an die europäischen Behandlungsmethoden und an Medikamente zu gewöhnen. Die Eingeborenen waren anfangs abgeneigt, sich ärztlicher Behandlung zu unterziehen. Der Heiltultul konnte Leute dazu überreden, einen Arzt im Krankenhaus oder während seiner Inspektionsreisen im Dorf aufzusuchen. Neue Arsenpräparate erlaubten es den Ärzten, die wunderbare Wirkung westlicher Medizin bei der Behandlung der Framboesie zu demonstrieren. Bei der Bekämpfung von Wurmkrankheiten war in Thymol ein wirksames und billiges Mittel erhältlich. Beide Leiden waren weit verbreitet aber nur selten lebensbedrohend, eigneten sich jedoch für Massenbehandlung. Eine Massenbehandlung für

Malaria, die viel gefährlichere Krankheit, mußte aufgegeben werden, da keine einfache, wirksame und zugleich billige Methode vorhanden war.

Bald nach dem Beginn der deutschen Kolonisation glaubte man, einen Rückgang der Bevölkerung feststellen zu können. Kämpfe zwischen Eingeborenenstämmen und niedrige Kinderzahlen wurden als Hauptgründe des Rückgangs betrachtet, doch kam man zur Überzeugung, daß die Befriedung der Volksstämme zusammen mit dem Einfluß der Missionen die Kämpfe und damit den Menschenverlust reduzierten. Das Problem der niedrigen Geburtenrate war komplizierter. Geburtenkontrolle, Kindertötung, jahrhundertelange Inzucht, Geschlechtskrankheiten und mangelnde Hygiene trugen alle zur niedrigen Kinderzahl bei. Verwaltung, Missionare und Plantagenbesitzer waren sich einig, daß aus moralischen und ökonomischen Gründen indigene Bräuche, die die Kinderzahl reduzierten, erst einmal ausgerottet werden müßten.

Rassenhygienische Theorien, die in Deutschland diskutiert wurden, fanden auch in Deutsch-Neuguinea Anklang, aber Experten waren über eine Degeneration der Melanesier, die sich anscheinend in einer Verminderung der Lebenskraft des Volkes manifestierte, geteilter Meinung. Einige nahmen an, daß sie einen unvermeidlichen und unaufhaltsamen Vorgang beobachteten; andere glaubten, daß die durch die Kolonisation erreichte Pazifizierung der Bevölkerung zu einem größeren Verkehr unter den Stämmen und damit zu einer natürlichen Blutauffrischung führen würde.

Ärzte sahen einen klaren Zusammenhang zwischen Arbeiteranwerbung und der Inzidenz der Geschlechtskrankheiten; der Zusammenhang zwischen Geschlechtskrankheiten und Bevölkerungsrückgang war weniger offensichtlich. Trotzdem war es unbestritten, daß diese Krankheiten bekämpft werden mußten. In Neumecklenburg, einem Gebiet, in welchem die Anwerbung von Männern und Frauen zur Plantagenarbeit schon in den 1880er Jahren üblich geworden war, waren Geschlechtskrankheiten besonders weit verbreitet. Daher wurde in Namatanai ein, in erster Linie für die lokale Bevölkerung bestimmter, ärztlicher Dienst eingerichtet. Außer dem Bau eines Eingeborenen-Krankenhauses wurde dort auch ein Arzt eingesetzt. Theoretisch war es seine Aufgabe, nicht nur im Krankenhaus zu arbeiten, sondern sich auch als Wanderarzt um die Gesundheit der Eingeborenen in den umliegenden Dörfern zu bemühen. In der Praxis verbrachte er jedoch die meiste Zeit im Spital.

Bei Kriegsausbruch hatte die Kolonialverwaltung relativ gute Kenntnisse über den allgemeinen Gesundheitszustand der Bevölkerung. In den Dörfern waren ärztlicherseits weitgehende Untersuchungen der Bevölkerung gemacht worden. Der dabei ursprünglich von der Verwaltung zur Verbesserung der

Volksgesundheit gewählte Weg war der Weg der Therapie. Öffentliche Arbeiten, wie z.B. die Wasserversorgung für Dörfer im Kampf gegen die Ruhr oder die Einschüttung naheliegender Sümpfe zur Verminderung der Moskitobrutstätten, wurden kaum unternommen. Der Vorschlag, die Frauenanwerbung in Neumecklenburg zu verbieten, stieß auf den Widerstand der Plantagenunternehmer und war politisch nicht durchsetzbar.

Mit der Ankunft von Dr. Wilhelm Külz im Oktober 1913, der vorgesehen war die neu geschaffene Stelle des Oberarztes für das Gesundheitswesen der Kolonie nach Vollendung der demographischen Forschung zu übernehmen, öffnete sich jedoch die Möglichkeit, den bislang eingeschlagenen Weg zu modifizieren. Seine frühere Tätigkeit als Regierungsarzt in den deutsch-afrikanischen Kolonien bestärkte ihn in seiner Meinung, daß in einem Kolonialstaat gesunde Kinder aufgezogen werden mußten, um dem stets wachsenden Arbeiterbedarf zu genügen. Andererseits hatte er aber beobachtet, daß koloniale Tätigkeiten für Eingeborenenvölker negative Folgeerscheinungen hatten. Solche, wie der Mangel an Hygiene und die von außen eingeführten Krankheiten, wirkten sich schädlich auf die Volksgesundheit aus. Gesundheitsprobleme waren nicht allein die Folge von bakteriologischen Krankheitserregern, sondern auch die Folge sozialer, ökonomischer und ökologischer Veränderungen. Seine Fragestellung richtete sich nicht so sehr auf den Rückgang der Bevölkerung, sondern auf die Möglichkeiten einer Bevölkerungszunahme. Seiner Ansicht nach sollte sich die öffentliche Gesundheitspflege vor allem auf die Dörfer konzentrieren, ganz besonders auf die Gesundheitsfürsorge für Frauen und Kinder. Nur gesunde Mütter konnten gesunde Kinder gebären und aufziehen. Hygienische Vorrichtungen, wie eine zuverlässige Wasserversorgung zusammen mit einem ärztlichen Dienst in den Dörfern, waren in seinen Plänen für die Volksgesundheit vorrangig.

Diese Politik fand in Deutschland Befürworter und so wurden vom Reichstag auch mehr Mittel bewilligt, um die Gesundheitspflege in den Dörfern zu verankern. Das Grundmotiv dabei war die totale Abhängigkeit der Kolonialunternehmer von ihren eingeborenen Arbeitskräften. Gesundheit war ein ganz enger Begriff, der sich auf die körperliche Fähigkeit für Plantagenarbeit und das Aufziehen einer großen Familie beschränkte. Die ganze Bevölkerung mußte gesund sein, um den zukünftigen Arbeiterbedarf zu decken und um Deutsch-Neuguinea in eine florierende Kolonie zu verwandeln.

Wie weit diese Erwartungen sich erfüllen konnten, bleibt Spekulation. Der Ausbruch des Krieges beendete das Experiment Deutsch-Neuguinea und neue Erfahrungen mit dem Gesundheitswesen konnten nicht mehr gemacht werden.

APPENDICES

APPENDIX I

Doctors in Kaiser-Wilhelmsland and the Bismarck Archipelago, 1886-1914

This list comprises all doctors who were employed as company or government medical officers from 1886-1914. Names marked # indicate a temporary appointment only while awaiting the arrival of a new doctor. (Frobenius worked for the Rhenish Mission, but acted several times as locum.)

Name	Arrival	Place/s of work	Departure
Schellong	28 Jan 1886	Finschhafen	April 1888
Lukowicz	9 April 1888	Finschhafen	March 1889
Herrmann	5 April 1889	Finschhafen	1889
Weinland	July 1889	Finschhafen	died 12 March 1891
Frobenius#	July 1890	Stephansort / FWH	1900
Emmerling	22 June 1891	Stephansort / FWH	died 20 Feb 1893
Hagge	early 1891	Stephansort	1893
Jentzsch	2 June 1893	FWH	April 1894
Hagen	12 Nov 1893	Stephansort	January 1895
Wendland	16 August 1894	FWH/Stephansort/	January 1898
	27 Nov 1901	Herbertshöhe	*(5 June 1915 ex Sydney)?
Dempwolff	9 March 1895	FWH	February 1897
	17 Oct 1901	Stephansort/ H'höhe	June 1903
Danneil	Jan.1896	Herbertshöhe	January 1899
	early 1904	Kaewieng/Rabaul	April? 1908
Diesing	Nov.1897	FWH	September 1898
Liese#	Sept 1898	Stephansort	April 1899
Fuhrmann	Jan.1899	Herbertshöhe	February 1901
Schlafke	Feb 1899	Stephansort	January 1900
Ollwig#	Jan 1900	Stephansort	June 1900
Jacobs	15 June 1900	Stephansort	June 1901
Hintze	23 April 1901	FWH	24 April 1902
Hoffmann	6 August 1902	FWH/Kaewieng	13 April 1914
Seibert	16 Feb 1905	H'höhe/FWH/Rabaul	17 May 1907
Runge	June 1906	FWH/Kaew./ H'höhe	*(13 March 1915 ex Sydney)
Born	end 1907	FWH/Rabaul/ H'höhe	end 1909
Wick	24 Oct 1908	Rabaul	*(13 Feb. 1915 ex Sydney)
Liesegang	April 1910	FWH	*15 March 1916
Kopp	1910	Kaewieng/Rabaul	January 1913
Kröning	13 Oct. 1911	Namatanai/Kieta	*(13 Feb. 1915 ex Sydney)
Kersten	24 July 1912	FWH/Rabaul	*15 July 1915
Braunert	30 March 1913	Namatanai	*(16 Jan. 1915 ex Sydney)
Külz	11 Oct 1913	Rabaul	* ?
Dieterlen	5 April 1914	Kaewieng	*(13 March 1915 ex Sydney)

* working in German New Guinea at outbreak of war in August 1914

APPENDIX II

Biographical notes on doctors in Kaiser-Wilhelmsland and the Bismarck-Archipelago, 1886-1914 (in alphabetical order)

Born, Walter, worked first on Yap as government medical officer. On returning from home leave at end of 1907 he was briefly sent to Friedrich-Wilhelmshafen, then to Herbertshöhe. He undertook a trip to Namatanai district from 22 February to 10 May 1908 to examine the health of indigenous population. From 15 May to 1 September 1908 he worked in Rabaul as locum, then in Herbertshöhe to the end of 1909. He was a very energetic and enterprising doctor; perhaps difficult to work with—the medical orderly wanted to resign two weeks after Born took up work, but the station manager persuaded him to change his mind. Early 1910 Born transferred to Jaluit, where he worked until end of November 1913; then to Truk—where he was still working in July 1914—to replace Mayer during the latter's home leave. By initiating the *Heiltultul* system, Born contributed more than any other doctor to the development of health services for the native population.

Braunert, Maximilian, on Jaluit from 1 February 1912 to early 1913. He transferred to Namatanai on 30 March 1913 and was still there when war broke out. Inflamed by patriotic fervour and alcohol, he was the "absolute ringleader" in the attack on Missionary Cox in Namatanai on 26 October 1914 and was sentenced to 30 strokes flogging, together with his more or less willing companions in crime, Hornung, Philipps, Koster and Paul. The flogging by Australian military authorities was carried out 30 November 1914, followed by immediate deportation on SS *Morinda*. Issued with a safe-conduct letter, he left Australia on 16 January 1915 on SS *Sonoma* for San Francisco to return to Germany. As a consequence of the flogging, all remaining German government employees—both senior government officials and doctors—resigned and were deported from New Guinea. Much to the embarrassment of the Australian government, the zealous dispensing of justice to German subjects by the Administrator, Colonel Holmes, turned into a minor international incident.

Danneil, Kurt, worked in Herbertshöhe as New Guinea Company doctor from January 1896 to January 1899. He returned to German New Guinea early in 1904 to take up an appointment as government medical officer in Kaewieng. In February 1908 he took up work in Rabaul, after returning from home leave; it is unclear what happened, but Dr. Born was recalled from Namatanai to work in Rabaul in May 1908; no further trace of Danneil.

Dempwolff, Otto (born 25 May 1871, died 27 November 1938). After two trips to South America as a ship's doctor, he worked for the New Guinea Company in Friedrich-Wilhelmshafen from 9 March 1895 to February 1897. In 1899 he joined the Colonial Troops and worked in Southwest Africa, then in Berlin in the Colonial Department, from where he was seconded to continue malaria research in New Guinea. He arrived in Friedrich-Wilhelmshafen on 17 October 1901. During his stay there he also took care of the New Guinea Company medical services in Stephansort from 17 May to 21 July 1902. Until June 1903 he was based in Herbertshöhe from where he made trips to the Western Islands (Wuvulua, Hermit and Ninigo island groups) and then returned to Germany. After his return to Germany, he worked for some months at the Institute for Infectious Diseases in Berlin. Then another tour of duty in Southwest-Africa and one in East Africa. Wherever he was working, he learnt local languages (mainly with the help of missionaries) and recorded information on these languages. On discharge from the Colonial Troops, he worked and studied at the Hamburg Kolonialinstitut. He returned to New Guinea for further linguistic studies early in 1914. He published a number of medical articles, especially on his malaria investigations, but his fame rests on his linguistic work, his research on Bantu and other African languages, and especially on Austronesian languages, for which he laid the foundations for all subsequent comparative work on their phonology and lexicon. Deported from Rabaul on 1 November 1914 on HMAS *Berrima*; issued with a safe-conduct letter, he left Australia on 16 January 1915 on SS *Sonoma* for San Francisco to return to Germany.

Diesing, started work in November 1897 in Friedrich-Wilhelmshafen as the successor to Wendland. Left in September 1898 because of disagreements with company management. Later he worked in Cameroon.

Dieterlen, Fritz, (military doctor, ex-Colonial Troops, seconded as government medical officer), arrived on 5 April 1914 to replace Hoffmann in Kaewieng; he resigned on 10 December 1914 and was taken to Rabaul as prisoner of war on 26 December 1914. He was deported from Rabaul on SS *Matunga* on 4 January 1915. Issued with a safe-conduct letter, he left Australia on 13 February 1915 on SS *Ventura* for San Francisco to return to Germany.

Emmerling, Philipp, (father senior government official in Darmstadt) ex-military medical officer, arrived on 22 June 1891. On the way to German New Guinea he spent some time in Java studying tropical medicine; he worked in Stephansort and Friedrich-Wilhelmshafen. He died there on 20 February 1893 of "fever and nephritis".

Frobenius, Wilhelm, (born 24 June 1855, in Bavaria; died 1927) arrived in July 1890 as a missionary doctor for the Rhenish mission, after having spent some time on Java in order to study tropical medicine. Although based with the mission, he regularly acted as locum in Stephansort, and assisted the resident doctor with operations or during times of emergency, such as the influenza epidemic in 1890/91. He married while on home leave in 1897 and returned with his wife to set up a new station on Bilibili in 1898. Left New Guinea in 1900 because of illness in his family; worked in Germany in the Bethler Anstalt, a charitable hospital.

Fuhrmann, M., worked in Herbertshöhe as New Guinea Company doctor from January 1899 to February 1901 and left on expiry of his contract.

Hagen, Bernhard, arrived in Stephansort on 12 November 1893. He had worked in Sumatra for 13 years before taking up an appointment with the New Guinea Company. Because of his experience in the tropics and with Malay and Chinese labourers, high hopes were held that he would be able to provide effective treatment of beriberi. He left in January 1895 for a convalescence trip to Sumatra, but as his health did not improve there, he returned to Germany. Published his memoirs *Unter den Papua's* in 1899.

Hagge, Reinhart, (aged 32) arrived early 1891 and worked for the Astrolabe Company in Stephansort. He left probably in 1893.

Herrmann, Eugen, (from Berleburg, Westphalia) arrived in Finschhafen on 5 April 1889, "a very highly recommended army doctor". He had serious disagreements with the management of the New Guinea Company which led to his dismissal. On the basis of his contract Herrmann did not consider himself to be subordinate to the director and was taken to court because of neglect of contractual duties. He refused to pay the fine imposed by the High Court in a hearing after his departure and the New Guinea Company sought to collect the fine through the courts in Surabaya, where Herrmann had taken up work after his departure from Finschhafen.

Hintze, Kurt, (born in Hamburg), had worked in Central America for some years; he attended courses at the Hamburg and the Berlin institutes. He was recommended to the New Guinea Company by Professor Koch and worked in Friedrich-Wilhelmshafen from 23 April 1901 to 24 April 1902, when he left because of ill health. Later he worked in Togo.

Hoffmann, Willy, took up work in Friedrich-Wilhelmshafen as New Guinea Company doctor on 6 August 1902 to replace Hintze. Although he had no tropical experience he was employed because of the urgent need for a doctor in Friedrich-Wilhelmshafen. He turned out to be a good choice, and when the government took over medical services for Kaiser-Wilhelmsland, he was appointed government medical officer. He worked there until 1910 and, following home leave, took up an appointment as government medical officer in Kaewieng in April 1911. He married Martha Ninehuch, a nurse working in Friedrich-Wilhelmshafen, in October 1910. Together with his wife he left New Guinea on 13 April 1914. He was a member of the German Society for Tropical Medicine.

Jacobs, G., attended a training course at the Institute for Infectious Diseases in Berlin before going to New Guinea (equipped with a Zeiss microscope). He worked in Stephansort from 15 June 1900 to 14 June 1901, when he left because of blackwater fever.

Jentzsch, Carl, started work in Friedrich-Wilhelmshafen on 2 June 1893 and left in about April 1894.

Kersten, Hans Ewald, began work in Friedrich-Wilhelmshafen 24 July 1912 as locum during Liesegang's home leave. He transferred in August to Rabaul 1913 where he was still working at the outbreak of war. He married Carla Hass-Merckel on 29 December 1913 in Rabaul; a daughter Liese was born at Gunantambu on 29 May 1915; he left Rabaul on SS *Marsina* together with wife and child in June 1915. He published a number of articles in *ASTH* on population surveys in Morobe district and Duke of York group. He was a member of the German Society for Tropical Medicine.

Kopp, Karl, arrived in New Guinea in 1910 as a member of the German-Dutch Border Expedition, and remained in the country after the conclusion of the expedition, first in Kaewieng to April 1911, then in Rabaul. From mid-October to mid-November 1912 he undertook an examination of the indigenous people on the northwest coast of New Britain. Soon after his return he fell sick with malaria with heart complications; with his wife returned to Germany on sick leave in mid-January 1913. Apparently unfit to work in a malarial region, he took up work in Jaluit in November 1913, replacing Born.

Kröning, Bruno, arrived in German New Guinea 13 October 1911. After a trip to the Admiralty Islands he took up his appointment as government medical officer in Namatanai 13 November 1911. From March 1912 he was acting district officer during the district officer's home leave. He transferred to Kieta in February 1913, where he was also acting station manager for some months. In 1913 he married Frances, the daughter of John Highley and his wife Phoebe (a Samoan relative of Emma Kolbe); he was deported on SS *Matunga* from Rabaul with his wife and daughter on 4 January 1915; issued with a safe-conduct letter, they left Australia on 13 February 1915 on SS *Ventura* for San Francisco to return to Germany.

Külz, Ludwig, worked in Togo from 1902 to 1905, and in Cameroon from 1905 to 1912. He arrived in Rabaul 11 October 1913 as senior government medical officer to implement new health care policies for the indigenous population. His first task, as a member of the medico-demographic research team, was to investigate the health status of the indigenous population in German New Guinea, with particular emphasis on the question of population decline. His research tour started off in Yap in November 1913. From there he went to the Gazelle-Peninsula, then to Kaiser-Wilhelmsland, and back east to New Ireland; he arrived in Kaewieng 19 July 1914. It is not clear how much work he did in New Ireland. The news of the outbreak of war reached him probably at Kaewieng. His name does not appear on any shipping lists and he may have made his own way back to Germany as has been suggested by Eckart. This, however, seems rather odd, as under the terms of capitulation agreed between Acting Governor Haber and Colonel Holmes, German officials were permitted to return to Germany with a letter of safe-conduct.

Liesegang, Fritz, (military doctor, formerly in German Southwest Africa). Working in Friedrich-Wilhelmshafen from 11 April 1910, he was on home leave for the first half of 1913 and returned with his wife 27 July 1913. A son was born in Friedrich-Wilhelmshafen 23 March 1914. Liesegang was still working in Friedrich-Wilhelmshafen when war broke out. He left Rabaul on SS *Matunga* on 18 March 1916, together with his wife and son. He was a member of German Society for Tropical Medicine.

Lukowicz, C.Z.M. von, studied medicine in Halle, graduated 1885; arrived in Finschhafen 9 April 1888 and worked there to end of March 1889. He did not complete his three-year contract, but the reasons for his early departure cannot be established. In all probability he went to Australia as he registered as medical practitioner in Adelaide, S.A., 3 December 1891.

Ollwig, Heinrich, (1836-1914) was an ex-military doctor and arrived as a member of Professor Koch's malaria research team. He worked as locum in Stephansort from January to June 1900, virtually the whole of Koch's sojourn in New Guinea, until a replacement for Schlafke arrived.

Runge, Hermann, arrived in German New Guinea in June 1906 and worked as locum in Friedrich-Wilhelmshafen. He then transferred to Kaewieng and, on return from home leave with his wife Lili (from 5 January - 13 October 1911), started work in Herbertshöhe, where he was still working at the outbreak of war. He trained as a dentist during 1911 home leave. Issued with a safe-conduct letter, he left Australia on 13 March 1915 on SS *Sonoma* for San Francisco to return to Germany. He was a member of German Society for Tropical Medicine.

Schellong, Otto, (born 13 May 1858 in Löbau, West Prussia; died in Königsberg on 13 February 1945; father clergyman). He studied at Koch's Institute for Infectious Diseases in Berlin for a brief period before departure for New Guinea. He arrived in Finschhafen 28 January 1885 and remained there to end of his contract; he left 17 April 1888. He was considered an expert on tropical medicine; he was also a collector of ethnographica and wrote extensively on New Guinea from a medical and anthropological point of view, and also on the labour question. His collection of forty plaster casts of people from Kaiser-Wilhelmsland and Bismarck Archipelago was sold to the Berlin Anthropological Society.

Schlafke, Anton, worked in Stephansort from February 1899 to January 1900 when he was diagnosed as suffering from tuberculosis by Professor Robert Koch and sent home. He died in Germany within a year of returning from New Guinea.

Seibert, Josef (born 9 March 1866 in Bensheim, Hessen, died 1930; father school teacher). After completing studies at the Berlin Institute for Infectious Diseases and the Hamburg Institute of Tropical Medicine, he arrived in Herbertshöhe on 16 February 1905 and worked as locum for Wendland until February 1906; then he spent a few weeks in Friedrich-Wilhelmshafen. He took up work in Rabaul as government medical officer in June 1906. Clearing and building work for the new station had begun and soon he began battle with the authorities about the generally poor working and hygienic conditions of the work force. He suffered a lot of ill health and was hospitalised in Herbertshöhe from 5 to 9 October 1905, from 10 January to 18 March 1906 and again from 9 April to 17 May 1907, when he left New Guinea to return home. He was a member of German Society for Tropical Medicine from its inception in 1907.

Weinland, Carl August Friedrich, (born 9 October 1864, near Urach, Württemberg, father zoologist) arrived in Finschhafen in July 1889 and died there of malaria on 12 March 1891, two days before the general evacuation. He was praised for "his energetic intervention" during an outbreak of cholera among the Chinese and Melanesian labourers in Hatzfeldhafen in November/December 1890. He had wide interests in ethnology and natural science; his collection of ethnographical, botanical and zoological (molluscs and helminths) materials went to German museums.

Wendland, Wilhelm, (born about 1867, father Mission Inspector for the Berlin Mission) took up his appointment as New Guinea Company doctor in Friedrich-Wilhelmshafen on 16 August 1894. He transferred for some time to the Astrolabe Company in Stephansort and, after returning to Friedrich-Wilhelmshafen, remained there until November 1897 when he was sent to Herbertshöhe to act as locum for Dr. Danneil who had been taken ill with dysentery. He returned to Germany early in 1898, then took up an appointment as government medical officer in Togo. On return to Germany in March 1901 he attended courses in tropical medicine at the newly opened Institute for Tropical Medicine in Hamburg. He left Germany again in September 1901 to take up his appointment as government medical officer in Herbertshöhe on 27 November 1901. According to his memoirs *Im Wunderland der Papuas* he he spent the next 14 years in Herbertshöhe and Rabaul, where he left "together with the last German government employees on S.S. *Matunga* " on 11 May 1915. According to the passenger list, the only German deportee was Judge Weber. If Wendland was also on this ship, it is likely that he left Australia on 5 June 1915 for San Francisco to return to Germany on SS *Ventura*, the ship on which Weber left with a safe-conduct letter. Salary records list him as having terminated government service at end of December 1913 and there is no further evidence of his presence in German New Guinea after that date in government files. It is however possible that Wendland set up a private practice in Rabaul. The government had been trying to encourage a medical practitioner to set up private practice in Rabaul since 1909. With contracts from private enterprise, a doctor would have a reasonable living, and it seems more likely that one familiar with conditions would set up privately, rather than a doctor from Germany with no colonial experience. He was a member of German Society for Tropical Medicine.

Wick, Willy, (born 1879, married, one daughter; was in Tsingtau from 1903 to 1907 as missionary doctor of Rhenish Mission). He studied at the Hamburg Institute of Tropical Medicine from 16 March to 21 May 1908. He took up work in Rabaul on 24 October 1908 as government medical officer; he returned from home leave 17 March 1913 and was working in Rabaul when war broke out. Together with his wife he appears to have been very active socially—they gave classical concerts at the Rabaul Club—and he applied for an alcohol licence for the Rabaul Club shortly after his arrival.

He published a few articles in *ASTH*. He was a member of German Society for Tropical Medicine. Issued with a safe-conduct letter, he left Australia on 13 March 1915 on SS *Ventura* for San Francisco to return to Germany. His wife and daughter left Rabaul on 9 June 1915 on SS *Matunga*, probably having stayed on to keep Mrs Kersten company during her pregnancy.

Sources: List compiled from details gathered in *NKWL* ; Annual Reports New Guinea Company; *Amtsblatt;* salary lists of imperial government; Colonial Office files; *Rabaul Gazette; DKB*; Australian Archives (ACT) records; *Pagel's Biographisches Lexikon;* Clasen, U., 1982, *Deutsche und deutschstämmige Aerzte in New South Wales und South Australia zwischen 1846 und 1911.*; W.U. Eckart, 1988, Medicine and German Colonial Expansion in the Pacific, in R. Mcleod, *Disease, Medicine and Empire*; S. Mackenzie, *The Australians at Rabaul*; T.D. Brock, *Robert Koch: A Life in Medicine and Bacteriology;* Blust, R. 'Dempwolff's Contributions to Austronesian Linguistics', *Afrika und Übersee* 71/2(1988): 167-76; Frau Duttge, personal communication.

APPENDIX III

Nurses in Kaiser-Wilhelmsland and the Bismarck Archipelago, 1891-1914

Name	Arrival	Place/s of work	Departure
Doetsch, Adele	1907?	FWH	1909?
Hertzer, Auguste	6 Feb 1891	FWH/ Stephansort/Rabaul	settled in Rabaul district1900 died there 1934
Hoffmann, Kunigunde	1912	Rabaul	?
Hunziker	?	Herbertshöhe	29 Oct. 1909
Jucknat, Johanna	13 July 1911	Rabaul	transf. FWH 11 Jan 1913 June 1913
Knigge, Mathilde	24 June 1892	FWH	discharged 1894 ill health
Kubanke, Emma	24 June 1892	FWH	1894
Lehfeldt, Charlotte	11 Jan 1913	Rabaul	*(13 Feb. 1915 ex Sydney)
Ludwig	1 Aug 1914	Herbertshöhe	*
Lux, Johanna	5 Jan.1911	Herbertshöhe	?
Meyer, Anna	1893	FWH	?
Müller, Ida	20 Oct 1909	Rabaul	21 Jan. 1913
Ninehuch, Martha	1909	FWH	married Dr. Hoffmann Oct.1910
Roevert, M.	13 July 1911	Rabaul?	?
Saul, Hedwig	23 June 1891	Stephansort	married
Schwieder, Margot	23 March 1912	Rabaul	*(13 Feb. 1915 ex Sydney)
Wagner, Therese	1904	Herbertshöhe	3 July 1910

* still in German New Guinea at outbreak of war in August 1914

This list is incomplete, but no further records available to complete listing

Biographical notes:

Hertzer, Auguste, arrived in Stephansort on 23 June 1891, together with Hedwig Saul. Hertzer had worked in German East Africa for some years, where in late 1889 her most famous patient was Emin Pascha (Eduard Schnitzer), the German doctor and adventurer. In German New Guinea her nursing was much praised by doctors and patients, and many are said to owe their life to her devoted and careful work. One of them was Governor Hahl, who suffered life-threatening attacks of blackwater fever in the first months of 1902. Hertzer herself suffered considerably from malaria and took convalescence trips to Java and Ponape.

In 1899 she moved permanently to the Gazelle Peninsula, where she bought a plantation property in Palaupai. Trained by Dempwolff in blood testing for malaria parasites, she screened the population on Matupi and in villages along Blanche Bay and the labour force in Rabaul for about eighteen months in 1902/03, and dispensed quinine. Her program, although successful, was discontinued because of lack of funds. She ceased work on the program to return to her property. She maintained close contact with other settlers, and took care of select patients, like Mrs. Hahl during and after childbirth. As her home town Graudenz became part of Poland as a result of the Versailles treaty, she was not expropriated and remained in New Guinea for the rest of her life. Auguste Hertzer died in Palaupai on 16 May, 1934.

Kubanke, Emma, arrived in Friedrich-Wilhelmshafen on 24 June 1892. She had trained at the Augusta-Hospital in Berlin. She suffered much ill health, but completed her contract and stayed there for two years. She never fully regained her health, and continued to suffer from effects of malaria for years; unable to take up nursing again, she was put in charge of a small home established in Berlin to provide temporary accommodation for nursing sisters organising their trip to the colonies and on returning for debriefing.

APPENDIX IV

Medical orderlies in Kaiser-Wilhelmsland and the Bismarck Archipelago, 1886-1914

Name	Arrival	Place/s of work	Departure
Altmann, E.	1892	Finschhafen	1897?
Bässler, R.	1892?	Stephansort	end 1892
Beck, L.	1894	FWH	?
Berg	1914	Rabaul	*
Boschat, C.	1887	Finschhafen/FWH	died 10 March 1900 FWH
Buhr	1907	?	?
Dahne, H.	1898	Herbertshöhe	?
Ewest	1906	Herbertshöhe/Kieta	* (13 Feb. 1915 ex Sydney)
Faulenbach	1907		* (13 March 1915 ex Sydney)
Girnus, F.	1913	Morobe/Kieta	* (13 March 1915 ex Sydney)
Gleichmann	1898	FWH	?
Gumbert	1910	FWH	?
Günther	1900?	Stephansort	?
Haecker	1899	Herbertshöhe	?
Hansen	1887	Finschhafen	died Oct. 1887
Hässelbarth	1911	Morobe	home leave May 1914
Hoek	1909	Kaewieng	?
Kapell	1906	Herbertshöhe/Rabaul	?
Kasten, A.	1895	FWH	1896
Kunth	1912?		?
Kunzmann	1893	Stephansort	?
Lachmann	1903	Herbertshöhe/Kaewieng	* (16 Jan. 1915 ex Sydney)
Lipphaus	1896?	FWH	1898?
Luhr	1912?		?
Manz	1913	Rabaul	accid. death March 1914
Martin	1886	Finschhafen	1887
Meerkatz	?	NGC,Herbertshöhe	*(4 Jan. 1915)
Mendelson	1889	Herbertshöhe/FWH	1892
Müller	1912?	FWH	?
Paul	1914	Namatanai	*(30 Nov. 1914)
Pulwer	1911	Rabaul/Manus	died 19 April 1912 Manus
Rannow	1892?	FWH	?
Reiter	1889	Finschhafen/FWH	1892 (ill health)
Schmidt	1891	Stephansort	?
Schumacher	1912	Manus	* (16 Jan. 1915 ex Sydney)
Schweighöfer	1894?	Stephansort	1896
Steinemann	1907	Eitape/Namatanai	?
Steinke	1905	Herbertshöhe/Rabaul	*
Ullrich	1914	Stephansort	*
Winkler	1899		?
Wocke	1908	Herbertshöhe/Rabaul	* (16 Jan. 1915 ex Sydney)
Woitschek	1899	Herbertshöhe/Rabaul	*
Wolfram	1913?	Morobe	*
Wostrack	1900?	Herbertshöhe/Namatanai	* (16 Jan. 1915 ex Sydney)
Wust	1914	FWH	*
Ziegler	1913		* (7 May 1915 ex Sydney)

* still in German New Guinea at the outbreak of war in August 1914; date of deportation in brackets

This list is incomplete, but no further records available

APPENDIX V

European Deaths in Kaiser-Wilhelmsland and the Bismarck Archipelago, 1887-1914

Year	Name	Age	Occupation	Place	Period in colony	Cause of death
1887	Claasen	45	stat.asst.	KWL		malaria
1887	Gemske		store mgr	KWL	9 mths	malaria
1887	Hansen		med. orderly	KWL	6 mths	malaria
1887	Nell		butler	KWL	11 mths	malaria
1887	Persieh	70	collector	KWL	recent	malaria
1887	Schleinitz (f)		Frau	KWL	6 mths	diphtheria
1887	Schlenther		stat.asst.	KWL	recent	malaria
1887	Vatan		missionary	BA	3 yrs	malaria
1888	Below		stat. mgr.	KWL		accidental drowning
1888	Berthelemy		stat. mgr.	KWL		mental disturbance
1888	Brunswick		trader	BA		unknown
1888	Hoppe		trader	BA		homicide
1888	Hunstein		stat. asst.	KWL		accidental drowning
1888	Laury		trader	BA		unknown
1888	Studzinka		trader	KWL		homicide
1888	Weisser		stat. director	KWL		malaria
1889	Bradley		trader	BA		homicide
1889	Eich (f)	39	missionary wife	KWL		malaria
1889	Hellwig		botanist	KWL	1.1 yr	dysentery
1889	Wackernagel		missionary	KWL		accidental drowning
1889	X01		trader	BA		homicide
1890	Arnold		gen. mgr.	KWL		malaria
1890	Coe		trader	BA		homicide
1890	Dörmann		stat.asst.	KWL		malaria
1890	Elske		stat.asst.	KWL		malaria
1890	Haas		trader	BA		homicide
1890	Jordan		govt. secr	KWL	3.3 yrs	TB (in Soerabaya)
1890	Pethke		stat.asst.	KWL		malaria?
1890	Poehlke		harbourm'r	KWL		malaria
1891	Apell	30	clerk	KWL	4 mths	malaria
1891	Bösch		missionary	KWL		homicide
1891	Brodscheit		s'visor	KWL		malaria
1891	child			KWL		malaria
1891	child [Kindt]			KWL		malaria
1891	Christer	28	clerk	KWL	8 mths	malaria
1891	Ermisch		policeman	KWL	2 yrs	malaria
1891	Gunderson		trader	BA		homicide
1891	Heins		seaman	BA		malaria
1891	Hermes		stat. mgr	KWL		influenza
1891	Hildebrandt	33	judge	KWL		malaria
1891	Hilger		clerk	BA		accidental drowning
1891	Höltig		stat.asst.	KWL		malaria
1891	Jäger		stat.asst.	KWL		malaria
1891	Koch		s'visor	KWL		influenza
1891	Langmaak		court offic.	KWL	2 yrs	malaria
1891	Langmaak		planter	KWL	1 yr	influenza
1891	Ludwig	30	store mgr	KWL		malaria
1891	Lutz		planter	KWL	7 mths	delirium
1891	May	25	clerical	KWL		malaria
1891	Moisy, v.		stat. mgr.	KWL	6 mths?	homicide

Year	Name	Age	Occupation	Place	Period in colony	Cause of death
1891	Müller		planter	KWL	3 mths	homicide
1891	Reckwerth	30	pr. secretary	KWL		malaria
1891	Ritzer		stat.asst.	KWL	7 mths	malaria
1891	Scheidt		missionary	KWL		homicide
1891	Weinland	27	doctor	KWL	8 mths	malaria
1891	Weller		ship's cpt.	BA		malaria
1891	Wissmann (f)		Frau	KWL		malaria
1891	Wissmann		gen. director	KWL		malaria
1891	X02		trader	BA		homicide
1892	Eich		missionary	KWL		malaria
1892	Erbleweit		engineer	BA		unknown
1892	Friedebach		missionary	BA	1 yr?	malaria
1892	Kras		missionary	BA	1 yr.	malaria
1892	Kunze (f)		missionary wife	KWL	1 yr	malaria
1892	Rohlack		administrator	KWL	1 mth?	malaria, heart failure
1892	Stalio		ship's captain	BA		homicide
1893	Arff		missionary	KWL		malaria
1893	Emmerling	31	doctor	KWL	1.8 yrs	malaria, nephritis
1893	Fenichel		missionary	KWL		unknown
1893	Schulz		carpenter	KWL	6 yrs	malaria
1893	X03 [Agatha?] (f)		missionary	BA		unknown
1893	X04		trader	BA		homicide
1893	X05		trader	BA		homicide
1893	X06		trader	BA		homicide
1893	Zander	38	trader	BA		suicide
1894	Helfer		missionary	BA	2 yrs	malaria
1894	Huser		missionary	BA	3 yrs	malaria
1894	Johannsen		engineer	BA		malaria
1894	Mendelson (f)		Frau	KWL		malaria;
1894	Nieters		missionary	BA	recent	malaria
1894	Rojahn		trader	BA		homicide
1894	Ruppert		missionary	KWL	2 weeks	malaria
1894	X07			KWL		unknown
1894	X08			KWL		unknown
1894	X09			KWL		unknown
1894	X10		trader	BA		homicide
1894	X11			BA		unknown
1894	X12			BA		unknown
1894	X13			BA		unknown
1895	Barkemeyer		missionary	KWL		malaria
1895	Ehler		explorer	KWL		homicide
1895	Piering	38	supervisor	KWL		homicide
1895	Schrader		Kaufmann	KWL	4 mths	malaria
1895	Vollprecht		plant. asst.	BA	2 yrs	malaria
1895	Wallenroth		planter	KWL	3 mths	dysentery
1895	X14		stat. asst.	KWL		malaria
1896	Chisholm		ship's cpt.	BA		alcoholism, heart failure
1896	Damm	29	technician	KWL		malaria
1896	Kärnbach	30	trader	KWL	10 yrs	liver disease
1896	Lehmann	27	supervisor	KWL		blackwater fever
1896	Schielkopf		trader	BA		homicide
1896	Vetter (f)		missionary wife	KWL		blackwater fever
1896	X15		child	BA		dysentery
1896	X16		trader	BA		homicide
1896	X17		trader	BA		homicide

Year	Name	Age	Occupation	Place	Period in colony	Cause of death
1897	Annert	30	trader	BA		homicide
1897	Beavis	37	trader	BA		homicide
1897	Clare	22	trader	BA		homicide
1897	Ernst [Benedicta] (f)		missionary	BA		unknown
1897	Hagen, v.	38	gen. dir. NGK	KWL		homicide
1897	Jensen?	49	trader	BA		malaria
1897	Kieft	44	missionary	BA		dysentery
1897	Krause	32	trader	BA		suicide
1897	Lang	27	trader	BA		malaria
1897	Pfeilmann	22	tradesman	BA		malaria
1897	Tindal	3	child	BA		malaria
1897	Wandres	9 m	baby	KWL		malaria
1898	Baumüller		stat. mgr	KWL	6 mths	malaria
1898	Knudsen		stat.asst.	KWL	1 yr?	unknown
1898	Kolshorn		ship's cpt.	BA		homicide
1898	Leonhardt			BA		homicide
1898	Müller		plant.asst.	KWL		blackwater fever
1898	X18 (f)		missionary	BA	5 mths	blackwater fever
1898	X19 (f)		missionary	BA	2.7 yrs	blackwater fever
1898	X20			BA	4 yrs	malaria
1898	X21			BA	4yrs	malaria
1898	X22			BA		TB
1898	X23			BA		dysentery
1899	Brennan	44	s'visor Fors.	BA		malaria
1899	Dathe	43	ship's capt.	BA	1.6 yrs	homicide
1899	Hanke (f)		baby	KWL		neonatal
1899	Hanke (f)		missionary wife	KWL		childbirth/malaria
1899	Hansen	32	trader	BA	6 yrs	hemoptysis TB
1899	Horz	29	carpenter	BA	9 mths	dysentery
1899	Johannsen	38	seaman	BA		homicide
1899	Klein	54	trader	BA	16 yrs	stroke
1899	Langmore	28	nil	BA	2 mths	TB
1899	Lindner	16	trader	BA	3 mths	malaria
1899	M[aetzke?]	30	trader	BA	2.3 yrs	homicide
1899	Roser [Dorothea] (f)	33	missionary	BA	2.7 yrs	blackwater fever
1899	Schulle	32	clerical NGK	KWL	1.3 yrs	malaria
1899	Steffen	29	s'visor	KWL	3 mths	malaria
1899	Voigt	26	ship's capt.	BA	2 mths	malaria
1899	X24		trader	BA		homicide
1900	Below	30	purser	BA	1.6 yrs	accidental shooting
1900	Boschat (f)		Frau	KWL	?	influenza, pneumonia
1900	Boschat		med. orderly	KWL	13 yrs	pneumonia, influenza
1900	Dunkel	37	merchant	KWL	12 yrs	malaria
1900	Nebe		missionary	KWL	6 wks	malaria
1900	Schleiermacher		missionary	KWL		malaria
1900	Spölgen		missionary	KWL		malaria
1900	Steussloff	29	govt. empl.	BA	5.6 yrs	blackwater fever
1900	Strassser	40	trader	BA	8 yrs	malaria
1901	Brillomet [Hilaria] (f)	28	missionary	BA	7.8 yrs	malaria
1901	Bruno		publican	KWL	2 yrs	heart failure
1901	Carlsbourn		trader	BA		homicide
1901	Carr	23	pr. secretary	BA	1 yr	homicide
1901	Dew [Aloisia] (f)	28	missionary	BA	6 yrs	pulm. TB
1901	Ehrlich	46	ship's capt.	BA		malaria, heart failure
1901	Genhichi	33	seaman	BA	transit	dysentery

Year	Name	Age	Occupation	Place	Period in colony	Cause of death
1901	Hansche		baby	KWL		malaria
1901	Held		missionary	KWL	3 yrs	malaria
1901	Lewerentz		clerk	KWL		suicide
1901	Loris (f)	35	missionary	BA	10 yrs	malaria
1901	Mencke	23	rentier	BA		homicide
1901	Schmidt	38	ship's capt.	BA	1.2 yrs	heart attack
1901	Schneider	34	trader	BA	6 yrs	blackwater fever
1902	Grey	48	accountant	BA	2 mths	alcoholism, heart attack
1902	Katz	24	planter	BA	1.3 yrs	blackwater fever
1902	Philippe [Damiana] (f)		missionary	BA	8.1 yrs	blackwater fever
1902	Roth	54	s'visor	BA		alcoholism, TB
1902	Wolff (f)	32	Frau	BA	7.3 yrs	homicide
1902	Wolff	4 mth	baby	BA		homicide
1902	X25			KWL		blackwater fever
1903	C[oe?]	26	trader	BA		pulm. TB
1903	Doehl			BA		homicide
1903	Eemeren	28	missionary	BA	6 weeks	appendicitis?
1903	F.	36	trader	BA	4 mths	liver cirrhosis?
1903	H.		trader	BA		drowned
1903	Howard	45	diver	BA	2 yrs	homicide
1903	J.	44	seaman	BA		alcoholism
1903	M.	27	missionary	BA	6 mths	malaria
1903	Reinhardt			BA		homicide
1903	W.	24	engineer	BA	1 yr	pneumonia
1903	X26		missionary	KWL		blackwater fever
1903	X27		missionary	KWL	1.9 yrs	malaria
1903	X28		exped.	KWL	1.3 yrs	blackwater fever
1904	Bley	29	missionary	BA	1 yr	homicide
1904	Buckley	43	trader	BA	20 yrs	unknown
1904	Dickens	24	settler	BA	3 mths	malaria
1904	Graham	33	trader	BA	1 yr	ruptured aneurysm
1904	Holbe (f)	23	missionary	BA	1.6 yr	homicide
1904	Horgren (f)	1	child	BA		cramps
1904	Kohn		empl. NGC	KWL		blackwater fever
1904	Parira	31	trader	BA		drowned
1904	Plaschaert	33	missionary	BA	3 yrs	homicide
1904	Rascher	36	missionary	BA	9 yrs	homicide
1904	Rath (f)	27	missionary	BA	5 mths	homicide
1904	Reimers		trader	BA		homicide
1904	Rondahl (f)	7	child	BA		encephalitis
1904	Rütten	31	missionary	BA	3 yrs	homicide
1904	Sacchi			BA	2 yrs	unknown
1904	Salka (f)	29	nun	BA	5 mths	homicide
1904	Schellkens	31	missionary	BA	5 yrs	homicide
1904	Schmidt (f)	24	nun	BA	5 mths	homicide
1904	T. (f)	3 mths	baby	BA		unknown
1904	Utich (f)	36	nun	BA	1.6 yr	homicide
1904	Weiher		plant.asst.	KWL	recent	accident
1904	X29		seaman NDL	KWL	transit	peritonitis
1904	X30		missionary	KWL		blackwater fever
1904	X31 (f)		missionary	KWL		blackwater fever
1905	A.	28	trader	BA	2.6 yrs	alcoholism
1905	B.	44	govt. empl.	BA	3 yrs	pneumonia, alcoholism
1905	D.	18	seaman	BA	1.3 yr	pulm. TB
1905	E.			BA		accidental drowning

APPENDICES

Year	Name	Age	Occupation	Place	Period in colony	Cause of death
1905	H.		settler	BA	3 mths	accidental drowning
1905	H.		settler	BA		accidental drowning
1905	L.	45	planter	BA	10 yrs	pulm. TB
1905	L.			BA		suicide, alcoholism
1905	M.	47	farmer	BA	2 mths	heart failure
1905	Niedt	32	missionary	BA	1 yr	accidental drowning
1905	S.			BA		homicide
1905	Winkler		missionary	BA	15 yrs	unknown
1905	X32	50?	farmer	BA	6 mths	heart collapse
1906	B.	42	settler	BA	1 yr	unknown
1906	D.	55		BA		unknown
1906	J.	35		BA		unknown
1906	J.	32	farmer	BA	1.6 yrs	blackwater fever
1906	K.	32		BA	8 yrs	cirrhosis of liver
1906	L.[Juliana?] (f)	29	missionary	BA	3.6 yrs	pulm. TB
1906	W. (f)	31	Frau	BA	2.6 yrs	pelvic peritonitis
1906	X33		clerk NGC	KWL		accidental drowning
1906	X34		seaman	KWL		blackwater fever
1907	B.	30		BA	6 weeks	malaria, heart failure
1907	B[erg?]	57	govt. empl.	BA	10 yrs	liver abscess
1907	Detleven	32	NGC empl.	KWL		accidental
1907	D[annbauer?]	27	missionary	BA	1.6 yrs	TB/meningitis
1907	Goutheraud	43	missionary	BA	19 yrs	TB
1907	I.	9 mth		BA		dysentery
1907	L.	29		BA	1.6 yrs	unknown
1907	Lieztke	28	collector	KWL		blackwater fever
1907	N.	40		BA	10 yrs	TB
1907	P.	18		BA	born GNG	pulm. TB
1907	S.3	22	seaman	BA	1.2 yrs	abscess of psoas
1907	Stehlin	29	missionary	BA	3 yrs	blackwater fever
1907	W.	28		BA	1 yr	suicide
1907	W. (f)	28		BA	1.6 yrs	blackwater fever
1907	X35		NGC empl.	KWL		blackwater fever
1908	B.	37		BA		suicide
1908	B[reckwoldt?]	18		BA	3 yrs	malaria
1908	C.			BA		unknown
1908	C. (f)	38		BA	6 mth	puerperal fever
1908	F.	30		BA		unknown
1908	J[kier?]	26		BA	4 yrs	blackwater fever
1908	K[uhn?]	47		BA		encephalitis
1908	P[arkinson]	23		BA	born GNG	suicide
1908	R.	52	planter	KWL		pulm. TB
1908	S[onnkalb?]	32	settler	BA	2 mths	malaria
1908	Stephan	36	doctor/expl.	BA	1 yr	blackwater fever
1908	W.	4		BA		unknown
1908	X36 [Simonis?] (f)		missionary	KWL		accidental drowning
1908	X37 [Mönch?]		child	BA		dysentery
1908	X38		collector	KWL		malaria and pneumonia
1908	X39		missionary	KWL		TB
1908	X40		empl. NGK	KWL		malaria
1908	X41	25	empl. NGK	KWL		blackwater fever
1909	D.			KWL		homicide
1909	F.	31		BA	3 mths	heart disease
1909	H.			KWL		blackwater fever
1909	H.		gold digger	KWL		heat stroke

213

Year	Name	Age	Occupation	Place	Period in colony	Cause of death
1909	H.		missionary	KWL		blackwater fever
1909	H.		missionary	KWL		blackwater fever
1909	L.	41		BA		homicide
1909	M.[argraff?]	44		KWL	17 yrs	chronic proctitis
1909	P. (f)	39		BA		childbirth
1909	P. (f)	3 days		BA		neonatal
1909	Parkinson	65	planter	BA	27 yrs	TB
1910	B.	22	seaman	BA		typhus
1910	B.	36	trader	KWL		accidental drowning
1910	B.	33	trader	BA	5 yrs	suicide
1910	C.H.	72	publican	BA	1 yr	arteriosclerosis
1910	G.		tourist	BA		accidental
1910	H. St.	41	ship's capt.	KWL	13 yrs	pneumonia
1910	H.E.G.	28	naval officer	BA		typhus, heart failure
1910	L.		trader	BA	7 yrs	accidental drowning
1910	L.W. (f)	39	missionary wife	BA	10 yrs	cancer
1910	O.	38	trader	KWL	7 yrs	accidental drowning
1910	O.A.	26	plant. asst.	BA	2 yrs	accidental
1910	Richards	46	hunter	KWL	21 yrs	homicide
1910	Sch.	23	seaman	BA		typhus
1910	Sch.	38	plant. asst.	KWL	13 yrs	suicide
1910	T.G.	61		BA	3.5yrs	unknown
1910	Th.J. (f)	61		BA	6 yrs	pneumonia
1910	X42			BA		pneumonia
1910	X43			BA		liver cirrhosis
1910	X44 (f)	29	nun	KWL		TB
1910	X45		missionary	KWL		liver abscess
1911	Drewske	26	seaman	BA	5 mths	accidental drowning
1911	Hansen	18		BA		pneumonia
1911	Hildebrandt	47	trader	BA	24 yrs	heart failure
1911	Hoffmann			BA		stillbirth
1911	Jeschke	33	missionary	KWL	5 yrs	blackwater fever
1911	Oeser	60	farmer	BA	5 mths	malaria
1911	Petersen	40	seaman	BA	16 yrs	ruptured spleen
1911	Peterson		hunter	KWL		homicide
1911	Scherer	27	missionary	KWL	2.6 yrs	kidney complaint
1911	Schultz		planter	KWL		unknown
1911	Wieners	42	trader	BA	19 yrs	blackwater fever
1912	Pulwer		med. orderly	BA	6 mths	dysentery
1912	Scharfenberger	35	missionary	KWL	7 yrs	heart complaint
1912	Weber, Er.		farmer	BA		homicide;
1912	Weber, Ew.		farmer	BA		homicide;
1912	X46			BA		suicide
1912	X47			BA		dysentery
1912	X48		seaman	BA		miliary TB
1912	X49			BA		pneumonia
1912	X50			BA		accidental drowning
1912	X51		child	BA		malaria
1912	X52			BA		stillbirth;
1912	X53 (f)			BA		heart attack
1913	X54			BA		accidental
1913	Boluminski	50	district officer	BA	19	stroke/heart attack
1913	Decker (f)		missionary wife	KWL	10 yrs	accidental drowning
1913	Decker		child	KWL		accidental drowning
1913	Decker		child	KWL		accidental drowning

Year	Name	Age	Occupation	Place	Period in colony	Cause of death
1913	Schnibbe		farmer	BA		blackwater fever
1913	Warnecke		govt. empl.	BA	14 yrs?	unknown
1913	X54		baby	BA		neonatal
1913	X55			BA		suicide
1913	X56			BA		appendicitis
1913	X58		seaman	BA		sepsis
1914	Arnthal (f)		tourist	BA		typhus
1914	Behn		plant. mgr	BA		unknown
1914	Breitenstein		missionary	BA	6 yrs.	accidental drowning
1914	Horgren (f)			BA		pneumonia
1914	Manz		med. orderly	BA	few mths	accidental
1914	Ruge		planter	BA		unknown
1914	Scharlauk	38	govt. empl.	BA	14 yrs	heart failure
1914	Schuster		DHPG	BA		unknown
1914	Wohlgemuth		mechanic	KWL		appendicitis
1914	X59			BA		stillbirth
1914	X60			KWL		blackwater fever

Glossary

X	no name
f	female
initial	only initial given in statistical reports
[...]	probable name of person

APPENDIX VI

Morbidity, European Hospitals, Herbertshöhe/Rabaul district, 1903-1911

Year	Total patients	A	B	C	D	E	F	G	H	I	J	K	L	M	N	O
1903	370	152	2	3	21	2	0	10	59	34	8	18	13	23	12	13
1904	259	106	0	6	13	1	0	7	33	40	7	6	3	20	14	3
1905	263	105	7	2	13	2	0	12	24	26	1	6	8	30	17	10
1906	305	108	1	3	14	5	0	12	35	46	3	5	27	19	16	11
1907	284	110	9	2	15	1	0	6	46	30	2	1	12	24	20	6
1908	359	100	7	2	34	0	0	27	63	37	5	13	17	33	17	4
1909	406	93	18	3	35	4	0	17	83	37	7	26	14	39	18	12
1910	478	127	7	2	28	4	0	21	98	54	5	27	11	51	26	17
1911	512	98	5	4	40	1	0	25	122	53	19	19	33	44	29	20

Key
A malaria and blackwater fever
B dysentery
C tuberculosis
D respiratory tract infections
E pneumonia and pleurisy
F beriberi
G venereal diseases
H general (includes heart, circulatory system)
I alimentary tract
J urinary tract
K eyes
L skin (tinea, rashes etc.)
M surgical (tropical ulcers etc.)
N injuries (cuts, contusions, fractures)
O gynaecological/obstetrics

Source: MB 1903/4-1911/12

APPENDIX VII

Morbidity, Government Native Hospitals, Herbertshöhe/Rabaul district, 1903-1911

Year	Total patients	A	B	C	D	E	F	G	H	I	J	K	L	M	N	O
1903	1032	209	2	0	68	10	10	14	45	14	0	18	102	402	137	1
1904	995	151	15	7	58	38	9	24	56	43	1	22	62	435	69	5
1905	999	191	83	8	62	13	20	71	41	22	20	8	53	348	50	9
1906	928	99	49	9	17	33	27	63	85	33	14	17	76	329	54	23
1907	673	143	24	13	32	27	25	42	72	27	11	15	32	159	36	15
1908	1261	239	86	13	65	81	16	74	101	115	11	35	40	321	40	24
1909	1928	263	153	13	68	37	34	155	115	101	32	92	96	681	82	6
1910	1701	173	63	26	25	37	50	235	261	86	31	110	9	489	77	29
1911	1537*	177	98	15	59	31	41	177	166	71	22	66	153	380	65	16

* in addition there were 553 cases of mumps

Key

A malaria and blackwater fever
B dysentery
C tuberculosis
D respiratory tract infections
E pneumonia and pleurisy
F beriberi
G venereal diseases
H general (includes heart, circulatory system)
I alimentary tract
J urinary tract
K eyes
L skin (tinea, rashes etc.)
M surgical (tropical ulcers etc)
N injuries (cuts, contusions, fractures)
O gynaecological/obstetrics

Source: MB 1903/4-1911/12

APPENDIX VIII

Hospitals in Kaiser-Wilhelmsland and the Bismarck Archipelago, 1887-1915

Year built or rebuilt	European Hospital	Native Hospital	Built by
1887	Finschhafen	Finschhafen	NGC
1889		Hatzfeldhafen	NGC
	Herbertshöhe		NGC
1891	Stephansort	Stephansort	NGC
1892	Friedrich-Wilhelmshafen	Friedrich-Wilhelmshafen	NGC
1896	Friedrich-Wilhelmshafen	Herbertshöhe	NGC
1901	Friedrich-Wilhelmshafen		NGC
1902		Herbertshöhe (1st stage)	GOVT
1904	Herbertshöhe	Herbertshöhe (2nd stage)	GOVT
		Friedrich-Wilhelmshafen	NGC
1906		Kaewieng	GOVT
1906		Herbertshöhe (3rd stage)	GOVT
1908		Friedrich-Wilhelmshafen (Isolation ward)	GOVT
1909		Rabaul	GOVT
1910		Namatanai (temporary)	GOVT
1911	Rabaul		GOVT
1912		Namatanai (1st stage)	GOVT
1913	Rabaul (2nd stage)	Manus (temporary)	GOVT
1914	Kaewieng (approved)	Friedrich-Wilhelmshafen	GOVT
		Kieta	GOVT
planned			
1915	Friedrich-Wilhelmshafen	Rabaul	GOVT
		Namatanai (2nd stage)	GOVT
		Kaewieng (Isolation ward)	GOVT
		Manus	GOVT
		Eitape	GOVT
		Morobe	GOVT

NGC = New Guinea Company

GOVT = Imperial government of German New Guinea

218

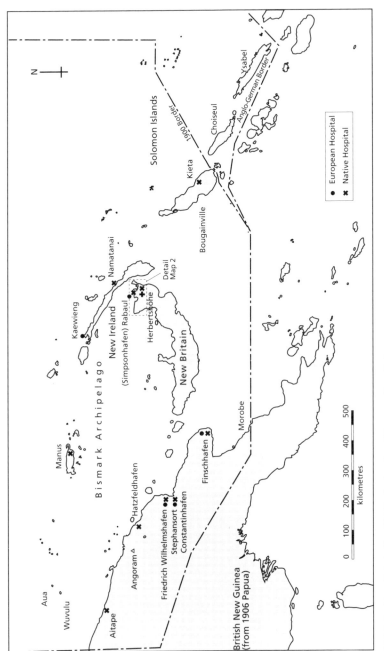

MAP 1. Hospitals in the Old Protectorate of German New Guinea

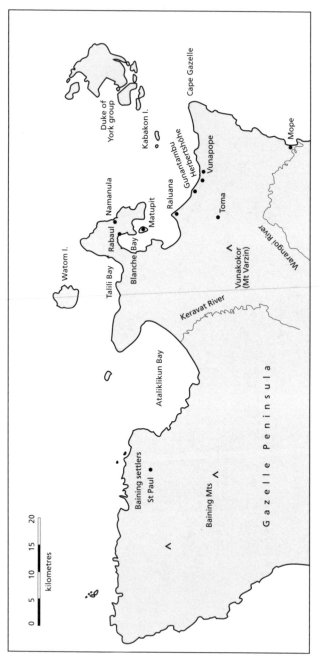

MAP 2. Northern half of the Gazelle Peninsula

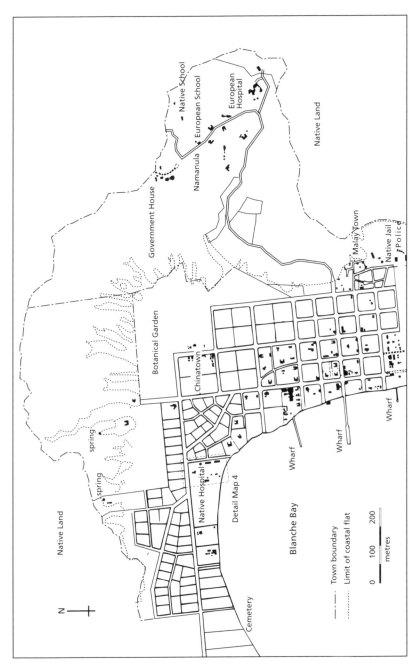

MAP 3.   Town of Rabaul, 1913

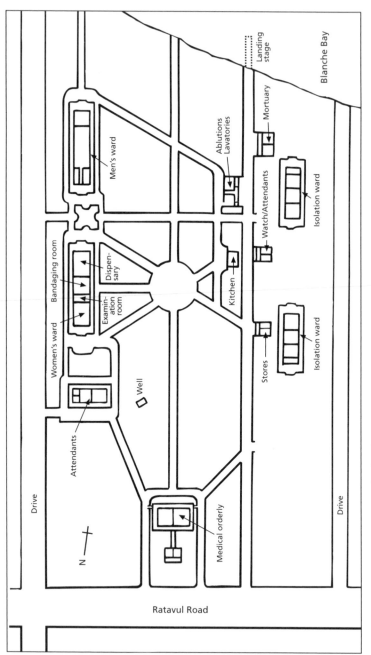

MAP 4. Sketchplan, Native Hospital Rabaul, 1909

BIBLIOGRAPHY

Unpublished Sources

Bundesarchiv, Abteilung Berlin - Reichskolonialamt Series (RKA)

2298-2314	Arbeiterfrage Neuguinea, 1884-1936
2392	Handels- und Erwerbsgesellschaften Neu Guinea, 1887-1933
2393-2394	Angriffe gegen die Gründungen der Firma W. Mertens & Co., 1907-14
2410, 2414	Beamte der Neuguinea Kompagnie, 1887-1901
2418-2420	Geschäftsberichte der Neuguinea Kompagnie, 1887-1910
2427-2429	Die Astrolabe Kompagnie, 1891-1897
2431	Die Firma Forsayth, 1899-1920
2535-2536	Opiumhandel, 1890-1914
2976-2996	Allgemeine Verhältnisse, Neuguinea, 1886-1915
4668-4669	Standesamt, Neu Guinea, 1888-1914
5729-5731	Krankenpflege im Schutzgebiet der Neu Guinea Kompagnie, 1896-1920
5769-5773	Gesundheitsverhältnisse in Deutsch Neuguinea, 1896-1930
5774	Gesundheitsverhältnisse Simpsonhafen, 1908-1909
5788	Gesundheitsverhältnisse Marshall-Inseln 1913-14
5802-5803	Gesundheitsstationen Neu Guinea, 1902-1914
5820	Apothekerwesen und Arzneihandel, Neuguinea, 1907-1914
5845	Malaria und Schwarzwasserfieber in Neuguinea, 1909-1910
5952	Massregeln gegen die Pest, Cholera und andere Epidemien, 1892-1920
6014	Medizinal-Jahresberichte 1910-1915
6045	Entsendung von Augenspezialisten nach Samoa und Saipan, 1909-1914
6047	Aerztliche Expedition Leber und Külz nach Neuguinea, 1913-1915
6512	Jahresberichte, Neuguinea, 1886-1892
7651	Fischerei, Neu Guinea 1899-1913

Government of Papua New Guinea, National Archives and Public Records Services

Records of the Imperial Government of German New Guinea, Series G254 and G255—
microfilms held by Australian Archives, ACT Regional Office, Mitchell, ACT

Australian Archives

Commonwealth Government Series CP 78/23 1489/72
Department of Defence Series MP 367/File 404/ll/52

Private Archives

Robert Koch Institut, Berlin
Bernhard-Nocht-Institut für Tropenmedizin, Hamburg

Private Collections

Private correspondence and papers relating to A. Engelhardt in the possession of Dr Berenwenger, Stuttgart, Germany
Private papers of Dr Dempwolff in the possession of Frau Duttge, Hamburg, Germany

223

Published Government documents

Amtsblatt für das Schutzgebiet Neuguinea. Rabaul. 1909-1914

Deutsche Kolonialgesetzgebung. Sammlung der auf die deutschen Schutzgebiete bezüglichen Gesetze. Berlin. 1893-1910

Deutsches Kolonialblatt. Amtsblatt für die Schutzgebiete in Afrika und der Südsee. Kolonial-Abteilung des Auswärtigen Amtes; Reichskolonialamt. Berlin: 1890-1914

German New Guinea: The Annual Reports, translated and edited by P. Sack & D. Clark. Canberra: Australian National University Press, 1979

German New Guinea: The Draft Annual Report for 1913-14, translated and edited by P. Sack & D. Clark. Canberra: Australian National University Press, 1980

Government Gazette, British Administration of German New Guinea. Rabaul. 1915

Medizinal-Berichte über die Deutschen Schutzgebiete. Kolonial-Abteilung des Auswärtigen Amtes, Reichskolonialamt. Berlin: 1905-1915; 1912/13 edited by Steudel, Beiheft 1, *ASTH* 28(1924)

Nachrichten über Kaiser-Wilhelms-Land und den Bismarck-Archipel. Neu Guinea Compagnie, Berlin (Ascher & Co.) 1885-1898

Stenographische Berichte der Verhandlungen des Reichstags, select volumes

Zusammenstellung der wichtigsten in DNG geltenden Erlasse, Verfügungen und Verordnung betr. den ärztlichen Dienst und das Gesundheitswesen. Rabaul 1913

Journals

Archiv für Schiffs-und Tropenhygiene (ASTH) 1897-1925

Barmer Missionsblatt, select volumes

Deutsche Kolonialzeitung (DKZ) 1884-1914

Berichte der Rheinische Missionsgesellschaft, select volumes

Die Katholischen Missionen, select volumes

Gott will es, 1903

Journal of Pacific History (JPH) select volumes

Papua New Guinea Medical Journal (PNGMedJ) 1966

Progenitor, 1987

Books, Articles and Dissertations

Contemporary Histories and Articles

Below. 'Bericht 66. Versammlung Deutscher Naturforscher und Aerzte, Sept. 1894', *DKZ* 11(1894): 145-7

—— 'Bericht 67. Versammlung Deutscher Naturforscher und Aerzte, Sept. 1895', *DKZ* 12(1895): 322-4

Besenbruch. 'Die Eingeborenenverhältnisse im Bezirk Nakanai', *Amtsblatt* 4(1912): 195-209, 243-48

Blum, H. *Neu-Guinea und der Bismarck-Archipel.* Berlin: Schoenfeldt & Co., 1900

—— *Das Bevölkerungsproblem im Stillen Weltmeer.* Berlin: Deutscher Verlag, 1902

Bögershausen, G. 'Die Augenkrankheit auf der Gazelle-Halbinsel', *Hiltruper Monatshefte* 4(1912)

Börnstein. 'Ethnographische Tätigkeit auf der Willaumez-Halbinsel', *DKB* 25(1914): 828-33

—— 'Forschungen auf den Admiralitätsinseln', *Petermann's Mitteilungen* 60 (I)(1914): 315-17

—— 'Ethnographische Tätigkeit auf Manus im Dezember 1913', *DKB* 26(1915): 154-61

Cohn, E. 'Zur Geschichte der Deutschen Tropenhygiene', *DKZ* 1(1900): 53-7

Dempwolff, O. 'Aerztliche Erfahrungen in Neu-Guinea', *ASTH* 2(1898): 134-300

—— 'Die Erziehung der Papuas zu Arbeitern', *Koloniales Jahrbuch* 11(1898): 1-14

—— 'Malariabekämpfung bei den Eingeborenen', *DKB* 15(1902): 201; 266

—— 'Bericht über eine Malaria-Expedition nach Deutsch-Neu-Guinea', *Zeitschrift für Hygiene und Infektionskrankheiten* 47(1904): 81-132

—— 'Ueber aussterbende Völker: die Eingeborenen der "westlichen Inseln" in Deutsch Neu-Guinea', *Zeitschrift für Ethnologie* 36(1904): 384-415

Deutsche Marine Expedition, Berichte (in 13 parts). *DKB*(1907 and 1908): 18 and 19

Dieterlen, F. 'Ueber eine im Jahre 1914 in der Südsee beobachtete Beriberi-Epidemie', *ASTH* 20(1916): 306-11

Eberlein, J. 'Nachrichten von St. Otto (Neu Pommern)', *DKB* 1(1899): 628-31

Friederici, G. 'Wissenschaftliche Ergebnisse einer amtlichen Forschungsreise nach dem Bismarck-Archipel im Jahre 1908', *Mitteilungen aus den Deutsche Schutzgebieten*, Ergänzungsheft Nr. 5, 1912

Fülleborn, F. 'Reisebericht über einen Besuch der tropenmedizinischen Schulen in England', *ASTH* 8(1904): 292-99

Giemsa, G. 'Trinkwasserverhältnisse und Trinkwasseruntersuchungen in den Kolonien', *ASTH* 7(1903): 447-55

—— 'Beitrag zur Frage der Stechmückenbekämpfung', *ASTH* 15(1911): 533-5

—— 'Das Mückensprayverfahren im Dienste der Bekämpfung der Malaria und anderer durch Stechmücken übertragbarer Krankheiten', *ASTH* 17(1913): 181-90

Hagen, B. *Unter den Papua's: Beobachtungen und Studien, Land und Leute, Thier- und Pflanzenwelt in Kaiser-Wilhelmsland.* Wiesbaden: Kreidel, 1899

Hahl, A. *Governor in New Guinea,* translated and edited by P. Sack & D. Clark. Canberra: Australian National University Press, 1980

Hirsch, A. *Handbuch der historisch-geographischen Pathologie.* Stuttgart, 1881

—— 'Acclimatisation und Colonisation', *Verhandlungen der Berliner Gesellschaft für Anthropologie, Ethnologie und Urgeschichte,* (Sitzung 27.2.1886) 1886: 155-66

Hoffmann, W. 'Ueber die Gesundheitsverhältnisse der Eingeborenen im nördlichen Neu-mecklenburg', *Amtsblatt* 5(1913): 114-31

Kersten, H.E. 'Bericht über Expedition nach Morobe', *Amtsblatt* 5(1913): 131-2

—— 'Die Sulka Siedlungen am St. Georgeskanal', *Amtsblatt* 6(1914): 213-7

—— 'Zur Frage des Bevölkerungsrückganges in Neupommern', *ASTH* 19(1915): 561-77

—— 'Die Tuberkulose in Kaiser-Wilhelmsland', *ASTH* 19(1915): 101-8

—— 'Die Gonorrhöe im Bezirk Rabaul', *ASTH* 29(1925), Beiheft 1: 180-5

Kimmle, ed. *Das Deutsche Rote Kreuz: Entstehung, Entwicklung und Leistungen der Vereinsorganisation seit Abschluss der Genfer Convention i.J. 1864.* 2 vols. Berlin: Boll & Pickardt, 1910

Koch, R. 'Third and fourth report on malaria expedition: German New Guinea', *British Medical Journal* 1900: 1183-86; 1597-98

—— 'Ueber die Bekämpfung der Malaria', *DKB* 11(1900): 943-47

—— 'Die Bekämpfung der Malaria', *Zeitschrift für Hygiene und Infektionskrankheiten* 43(1902): 1-4

Kohl, L. 'Die Verlegung des Gouvernements von Herbertshöhe nach Simpsonhafen', *Amtsblatt* 1(1909): 54-55

Kopp, K. 'Bericht über die Dysenterie-Bekämpfung in Manus', *Amtsblatt* 4(1912): 151-4

—— 'Zur Frage des Bevölkerungsrückganges in Neupommern', *ASTH* 17(1913): 729-50. Also translated as 'The native population of New Britain: do they decline? and what are the causes?' in *Government. Gazette, British Admininistration of German New Guinea* 2(1):8-12, 1915

—— 'Die Lebensaussichten der grossen Völkerschaften in Deutsch-Neuguinea, gemessen an der Proliferation', *Koloniale Rundschau* 1921: 119-26

Krieger, M. ed. *Neu-Guinea*. Berlin: Schall, 1899

Kuhn, P. 'Fortschritte der Tropenhygiene', DKZ 24(1907): 409-10

Külz, L. and Leber, A. 'Bericht der medizinisch-demographischen Südsee-Expedition über die Gazelle-Halbinsel', *DKB* 25(1914): 782-90

Külz, L. 'Der hygienische Einfluss der weissen Rasse auf die schwarze Rasse in Togo', *Archiv für Rassen- und Geschellschaftsbiologie* 2.4(1905)

—— 'Wesen und Ziele der kolonialen Eingeborenenhygiene', *ASTH* 14(1910): 651- 2 (also in *3. Kolonialkongress 1910*: 342-56. Berlin: Reimer)

—— 'Die Volkshygiene für Eingeborene und ihre Beziehung zur Kolonialwirtschaft und Kolonialverwaltung', *DKB* 21(1910): 12-21

—— 'Grundzüge der kolonialen Eingeborenenhygiene', *ASTH* 15(1911), Beiheft 8

—— 'Die seuchenhaften Krankheiten des Kindesalters der Eingeborenen und ihre Bedeutung für die koloniale Bevölkerungsfrage', *Koloniale Rundschau* 1913: 321-30.

—— 'Zur Pathologie und Demographie der Insel Jap, unter besonderer Berücksichtigung ihres Bevölkerungsrückganges', *DKB* 25(1914): 561-77

—— 'Zur Biologie und Pathologie des Nachwuchses bei den Naturvölkern der Deutschen Schutzgebiete', *ASTH* 23(1919): Beiheft 3

—— 'Ueber das Aussterben der Naturvölker. Ursachen und Verlaufsformen unter besonderer Berücksichtigung der Eingeborenen in den Deutschen Kolonien', *Archiv für Frauenkunde und Eugenik* 5.2/3(1919):114-44

—— 'Ueber das Aussterben der Naturvölker. Der Aussterbe-Mechanismus bei den Karolinern der Insel Jap', *Archiv für Frauenkunde und Eugenik*. 6.1(1920): 43-85

Leber, A. 'Centrale Durchquerung der Insel Manus (Admiralitäts-Inseln), Mai 1914', unpublished manuscript. Australian Archives, VIC, Department of Defence Accession MP 367, File No 404/11/52

Mayer, M. 'Tropenhygiene und Tropenkrankheiten auf der Internationalen Hygiene-Ausstellung zu Dresden', *ASTH* 15(1911): 785-89

Mense, C. 'Die Deutsche Tropenmedizin vor 25 Jahren und später', *ASTH* 25(1921): 2-13

Mühlens, P. 'Malariabekämpfung in Wilhelmshaven und Umgebung', *ASTH* 13(1909): 166-73

Neuhauss, R. *Deutsch Neu-Guinea*. 3 vols. Berlin: Dietrich Reimer, 1911

Nocht, B. 'Das neue Institut für Schiffs- und Tropenkrankheiten', *ASTH* 18(1914), Beiheft 5

Parkinson, R. *Dreissig Jahre in der Südsee*. Stuttgart: Stecker & Schröder, 1907

Plehn, A. *Kurzgefasste Vorschriften zur Verhütung und Behandlung tropischer Krankheiten*. Jena: Gustav Fischer, 1906

Plehn, F. *Tropenhygiene: Aerztliche Ratschläge für Kolonialbeamte, Offiziere, Missionare, Expeditionsführer, Pflanzer und Faktoristen*. Jena: Gustav Fischer, 1902

Ranke, C.E. *Ueber die Einwirkung des Tropenklimas auf die Ernährung des Menschen*. Berlin, 1900

Rascher, M. 'Auf der Suche nach Pocken', *Hiltruper Monatshefte* 1898: 229-34; 243- 48; 262-66

Ruge, R. 'Die Malariabekämpfung in den Deutschen Kolonien und in der Kaiserlichen Marine seit dem Jahr 1901', *ASTH* 11(1907): 705-18

Runge. 'Beriberifälle in Käwieng', *Amtsblatt* 1(1909): 138-40

—— 'Ueber sanitäre Eingeborenenfürsorge in Nord Neu-Mecklenburg', *Amtsblatt* 1 (1909): 143-44

Sander. 'Bericht 75. Versammlung Deutscher Naturforscher und Aerzte, September 1903', *DKZ* 20(1903): 403-5

—— 'Die erste Versammlung der Deutschen Tropenmedizinischen Gesellschaft in Hamburg', *DKZ* 25(1908): 292-3

Sapper, K. 'Bevölkerungsabnahme und Arbeiteranwerbung auf Neumecklenburg', *Amtsblatt* 1(1909): 176-8

—— 'Wissenschaftliche Ergebnisse einer amtlichen Forschungsreise nach dem Bismarck-Archipel im Jahre 1908' *Mitteilungen aus den Deutschen Schutzgebieten*, 1910, Ergänzungsheft 3

Schellong, O. 'Tropenhygienische Betrachtungen unter spezieller Berücksichtigung der für Kaiser-Wilhelmsland in Betracht kommenden Verhältnisse', *DKZ* 5(1888): 341-3, 363-4, 368-71

—— 'Ueber Familienleben und Gebräuche der Papuas der Umgebung von Finschhafen(Kaiser-Wilhelmsland)', *Zeitschrift für Ethnologie* 20(1888): 10-25

—— 'Der Deutsche in Kaiser-Wilhelmsland in seiner Stellungsnahme zum Landeseingeborenen', *DKZ* 6(1889): 69-70; 74-5; 85-6

—— 'Ueber Familienleben und Gebräuche der Papuas der Umgebung von Finschhafen (Kaiser-Wilhelmsland)', *Zeitschrift für Ethnologie* 21(1889): 10-25

—— 'Dreissig Thesen zur Diskussion der Malaria', *DKZ* 2(1889): 273-75

—— 'Beiträge zur Anthropologie der Papuas von Neu-Guinea (Nordost, Kaiser Wilhelms-Land)', *Zeitschrift für Ethnologie* 23(1891): 158-230

—— 'Das Tropenklima und sein Einfluss auf das Leben und die Lebensweise des Europäers', *Koloniales Jahrbuch* 5(1892): 58-67

—— 'Akklimatisation und Tropenhygiene' in T. Weyl, ed. *Handbuch der Hygiene*, Jena: G. Fischer, 1894

—— 'Tropenhygienisches', *DKZ* 14(1897): 64

—— 'Die Neu-Guinea Malaria einst und jetzt', *ASTH* 5(1901): 303-27

—— 'Mitteilungen über die Papuas (Jabim) der Gegend des Finschhafens', *Zeitschrift für Ethnologie* 37(1905): 602-18

—— *Alte Dokumente aus der Südsee: Zur Gründung einer Kolonie. Erlebtes und Eingeborenenstudien.* Königsberg: 1934

—— 'Die Anfänge und ersten Jahre deutscher Kolonisation in Neuguinea (Kaiser-Wilhelmsland)', *DKZ* 51(1939): 69-73; 91

Schilling, C. 'Der ärztliche Dienst in den deutschen Schutzgebieten', *ASTH* 13(1909), Beiheft 6: 32-45; also *DKB* 20: 966-70

—— 'Welche Bedeutung haben die neuen Fortschritte der Tropenhygiene für unsere Kolonien?', *3. Kolonialkongress 1910,* Berlin: Reimer, 1910

Schmidt, P. 'Ueber Anpassungsfähigkeit der weissen Rasse an das Tropenklima', *ASTH* 14(1910): 397-416

Schoen, E. 'Die Verhandlungen der Sektion Tropenhygiene', *DKZ* 14(1897): 414-5

Siebert, C. 'Ueber Wesen und Verbreitung von Haut- und Geschlechtskrankheiten in Nord-Neumecklenburg (Bismarck Archipel)', *ASTH* 13(1909): 201-14

Stephan E. & Graebner, F., eds. *Neu-Mecklenburg (Bismarck-Archipel). Die Küste von Umuddu bis Kap St. Georg, Forschungsergebnisse bei den Vermessungsfahrten von S.M.S.* Möwe *im Jahre 1904.* Berlin: Reimer, 1907

Stephan, E. 'Aerztliche Beobachtungen bei einem Naturvolke', *Archiv für Rassen- und Gesellschaftsbiologie* 5/6(1905): 799-811

Steudel, E. 'Kann der Deutsche sich in den Tropen akklimatisieren?', *DKB* 19(1908): 719-27

—— 'Der ärztliche Dienst in den Deutschen Schutzgebieten', *ASTH* 13(1909), Beiheft 6: 17-45; also *DKB* 20(1909): 921-26

Van der Burg. 'L'alimentation des Européens et des travailleurs indigènes aux pays chauds', *Janus* 10(1905): 88-94

Virchow, R. 'Acclimatisation', *Verhandlungen der Berliner Gesellschaft für Anthropologie, Ethnologie und Urgeschichte* (Sitzung 16.5.1885) 1885: 202-14

Wendland, W. 'Ueber das Auftreten der Beri-Beri-Krankheit in Kaiser-Wilhelmsland', *ASTH* 1(1897): 237-44

—— 'Ueber Chininprophylaxe in Neuguinea', *ASTH* 8(1904): 431-54

—— *Im Wunderland der Papuas: Ein deutscher Kolonialarzt erlebt die Südsee.* Berlin-Dahlen: Kurzeja, 1939

Wick, W. 'Ruhr: allgemeinverständliche Abhandlung', *Amtsblatt* 1(1909): 51-4

—— *Physiologische Studien zur Akklimatisation an die Tropen. ASTH* 14(1910): 605-16

—— 'Die gesundheitlichen Verhältnisse im mittleren Neumecklenburg', *Amtsblatt* 3(1911): 234-5. 240-1

—— *Besuch der Witu-Inseln. DKB* 25(1914): 97-98; also *Amtsblatt* 6(1914): 180-1

Ziemann, H. 'Wie erobern wir Afrika für die weisse und farbige Rasse?' *ASTH* 11(1907), Beiheft 5

—— 'Ueber die Errichtung von Tropeninstituten und die Gestaltung des ärztlichen Dienstes in den deutschen Schutzgebieten', *ASTH* 13(1909), Beiheft 6: 47-54 (Verhandlungen der deutschen tropenmedizinischen Gesellschaft, 2. Tagung, April 1909)

—— 'Tagung der Deutschen Tropenmedizinsichen Gesellschaft, April 1914', *DKZ* 31(1914): 280-2

Modern Histories and Articles

Ackerknecht, E.H. *Rudolf Virchow, Doctor, Statesman, Anthropologist* Madison: University of Wisconsin Press, 1953

Adams, M. B., ed. *The Wellborn Science: Eugenics in Germany, France, Brazil, and Russia.* Oxford: Oxford University Press, 1990

Allen, B.J. 'A Bomb or a Bullet or the Bloody Flux? Population Change in the Aitape Inland, Papua New Guinea, 1941-1945', *JPH* 18.3/4(1983): 218-235

Beck, Ann. 'The role of medicine in German East Africa', *Bulletin of History of Medicine* 45(1971): 179-8

—— 'Medical Administration and Medical Research in Developing Countries: Remarks on their History in Colonial East Africa', *Bulletin of the History of Medicine*, 46.4(1972): 349-58

Bell, C.O., ed. *The Diseases and Health Services of Papua New Guinea*, Port Moresby: Dept. of Public Health, 1973

Black, R.H. 'The Epidemiology of Malaria in Southwest Pacific', *South Pacific* 9.6(1957): 417-21

Blackburn, C.R.B. 'Medicine in New Guinea: three and a half centuries of change', *Postgraduate Medical Journal* 46(1970): 250-256

Blust, R. 'Dempwolff's Contribution to Austronesian Languages', *Afrika und Übersee* 71(1988): 167-76

Brock, T.D. *Robert Koch: A Life in Medicine and Bacteriology.* Madison: Science Tech Publishers; Berlin: Springer-Verlag, 1986

Bruce-Chwatt, L.J. *The Rise and Fall of Malaria in Europe.* Oxford: Oxford University Press, 1980

Burnett, Sir Macfarlane. *Natural History of Infectious Disease*, 2nd edition. Cambridge: Cambridge University Press, 1953

Burton-Bradley, B. G., ed. *A Medical History of Papua New Guinea: Vignettes of an earlier Period.* Kingsgrove, NSW: Australasian Medical Publishing Co. Ltd., 1990.

Burton, J. 'A Dysentery Epidemic in New Guinea and its Mortality', *JPH* 18.3/4(1983): 236-61

Dening, G. *Islands and Beaches: Discourse on a Silent Land, Marquesas 1774-1880.* Melbourne: Melbourne University Press, 1966

Davies, M. 'Das Gesundheitswesen im Kaiser-Wilhelmsland und im Bismarck-Archipel'. In H.J. Hiery, ed., *Handbuch der deutschen Südsee 1884-1914.* Paderborn: Schöningh Verlag, 2001

Denoon, D. with K. Dugan and L. Marshall. *Public Health in Papua New Guinea: Medical Possibility and Social Constraint, 1884-1984.* Cambridge: Cambridge University Press, 1989

Denoon, D. & C. Snowden, eds., *A Time to Plant and a Time to Uproot: A History of Agriculture in Papua New Guinea.* Port Moresby, Institute of Papua New Guinea Studies, 1981

Denoon, D. 'Temperate Medicine and Settler Capitalism: On the Reception of Western Medical Ideas', in R. Macleod, ed., *Disease, Medicine and Empire*, 121-138. London: Routledge, 1981

Eckart, W.U. 'Der ärztliche Dienst in den ehemaligen deutschen Kolonien', *Arzt und Krankenhaus* 10(1981): 422-26

—— 'Medicine and German colonial expansion in the Pacific.' In R. Macleod, ed., *Disease, Medicine and Empire: Perpectives on western medicine and the experience of European expansion*, 80-102. London: Routledge, 1988.

Evans, R.J. *Death in Hamburg: Society and Politics in the Cholera Years 1830-1910*. Oxford: Clarendon Press, 1987

Ewers, W.H. 'Malaria in the early years of German New Guinea', *Journal of the Papua and New Guinea Society* 6.1(1972): 3-30

Fanon, F. 'Medicine and Colonialism: The Algerian example', in J. Ehrenreich, ed. *The Cultural Crisis in Modern Medicine*, 229-51. N.Y.: Monthly Review Press, 1978

Firth, S. 'The New Guinea Company, 1885-1899: A Case of Unprofitable Imperialism', *Historical Studies* 15(1972): 361-77

—— 'The Transformation of the Labour Trade in German New Guinea', 1899-1914. *JPH* 11.1(1976): 51-65

—— *New Guinea under the Germans*. Melbourne: Melbourne University Press, 1982

—— 'German New Guinea: The Archival Perspective', *JPH* 20.2(1985): 94-103

Fischer, H. *Die Hamburger Südsee-Expedition: Ueber Ethnographie und Kolonialismus*. Frankfurt a.M.: Syndikat, 1981

Gann, L.H. & P. Duignan. *The Rulers of German Africa, 1884-1914*. Stanford: Stanford University Press, 1977

Gründer, H. *Geschichte der deutschen Kolonien, 3rd edition*. Paderborn: Schöningh, 1995

Hartwig, G.W. & K.D. Patterson, eds. *Disease in African History*. Durham, N.C.: Duke University Press, 1978

Headrick, D.R. 'Malaria, Quinine, and the Penetration of Africa', in his *The Tools of Empire*, 58-79. Oxford: Oxford University Press, 1981

Hempenstall, P. *Pacific Islanders under German Rule: A Study in the Meaning of Colonial Resistance*. Canberra. ANU Press, 1978

Herder, J. G. *Ideen zur Philosophie der Geschichte der Menschheit,* edited and annotated by H. Düntzer. Berlin: G. Hempel, no date

Heteren, G.M., van et al, eds.. *Dutch Medicine in the Malay Archipelago 1816-1942*. Amsterdam: Atlanta, 1989

Heyningen, E.B. van. 'Agents of Empire: the Medical Profession in the Cape Colony, 1880-1910', *Medical History* 33(1989): 450-471

Hiery, H.J. *Das Deutsche Reich in der Südsee 1900-1921. Eine Annäherung an die Erfahrungen verschiedener Kulturen*. Göttingen: Vandenhoeck & Ruprecht, 1995

—— *The Neglected War. The German South Pacific and the Influenmce of World War I*. Honolulu: University of Hawai'i Press, 1995

Hiery, H.J. and J.M. MacKenzie, eds. *European Impact and Pacific Influence. British and German Colonial Policy in the Pacific islands and the Indigenous Response*. London/New York: Tauris Academic Studies in association with the German Historical Institute London, 1997

Huerkamp, C. 'The History of Smallpox Vaccination in Germany', *JCH* 20(1985): 617-35

—— *Der Aufstieg der Ärzte im 19. Jahrhundert. Vom gelehrten Stand zum professionellen Experten: Das Beispiel Preußen*. Göttingen: Vandenhoeck & Ruprecht, 1985

Jackman, H.H. '*Nunquam otiosus* and the two Ottos: malaria in German New Guinea', in B.G. Burton-Bradley, *A History of Medicine in Papua New Guinea: Vignettes of an Earlier Period*, 119-150. Kingsgrove, NSW: Australasian Medical Publishing Co. Ltd., 1990

Jusatz, H. 'Wandlungen der Tropenmedizin am Ende des 19. Jahrhunderts', in G. Mann and R. Winau, eds. *Medizin, Naturwissenschaft, Technik und das Zweite Kaiserreich*, 227-38. (Studien zur Medizingeschichte) Göttingen: Vandenhoeck & Ruprecht, 1977

Kluxen, G. *Augenheilkunde Deutscher Tropenärzte vor 1918*. Düsseldorfer Arbeiten zur Geschichte der Medizin 5. Düsseldorf: Triltsch Druck und Verlag, 1980

Knoll, A.J. and L.H. Gann, eds,. *Germans in the Tropics: Essays in German Colonial History*. New York: Greenwood Press, 1987

Latukefu, S., ed., *Papua New Guinea: a Century of Colonial Impact 1884-1984*. Port Moresby: NRI and UPNG, 1989

Lea, D. & Lewis, L. 'Masculinity in Papua New Guinea', in L.A. Kosinski & J. Webb, eds., *Population at Microscale*, 65-78. New Zealand Geographical Society, 1976

MacLeod, R., & Lewis, M., eds., *Disease, Empire and Medicine: Perpectives on Western Medicine and the Experience of European Expansion*. London: Routledge, 1988

Mackenzie, S.S. *The Australians at Rabaul: The Capture and Administration of the German Possessions in the Southern Pacific. (Official History of Australia in the War of 1914-18*, vol. X) 4th edition. Sydney: Angus & Robertson Ltd., 1937

Maddocks, I. 'The Fruits of Malaria Control', *PNGMedJ* 10.2(1967): 33-4

—— 'Communicable Disease in Papua and New Guinea', *PNGMedJ* 13.4(1970): 120-4

—— 'Medicine and Colonisation', *Australian & New Zealand Journal of Sociology* 11.3(1975): 27-33

Moses, J. 'Imperial German Priorities in New Guinea 1885-1914' in S. Latukefu, ed., *Papua New Guinea: a Century of Colonial Impact, 1884-1984,* Port Moresby: NRI and UPNG, 1989

Parlow, S. 'Ueber einige kolonialistische und annexionistische Aspekte bei deutschen Aerzten von 1884 bis zum Ende des 1. Weltkrieges', *Wissenschaftliche Zeitschrift der Universität Rostock* (mathematisch-naturwissenschaftliche Reihe) 15.3/4 (1966): 537-49

Pierard, R.V. 'The German Colonial Society' in A.J. Knoll & L.H. Gann, eds., *Germans in the Tropics. Essays in German Colonial History*. New York: Greenwood Press, 1987

Radford, A.J., Speer, A. 'Medical Tultuls and Aid Post Orderlies: Some Historical Notes on the Use of Village Health Workers in Papua New Guinea up to Independence', *PNG Medical Journal* 29.2(1986): 166-88

Rowley, C.D. 'The Promotion of Native Health in German New Guinea', *South Pacific* 9.5(1957): 391-9. Melbourne: Melbourne University Press, 1958

Sack, P. & Clark, D., translators and editors. *Eduard Hernsheim: South Sea Merchant*. Boroko: IPNGS, 1983

Sack, P. 'a history of German New Guinea: a Debate about Evidence and Judgement', *JPH* 20.2(1985): 84-94

Scarr, D. *Fragments of Empire: A History of the Western Pacific High Commission 1877-1914*. Canberra: Australian National University Press, 1967

Scott, H.H. *A History of Tropical Medicine.* (two vols.) London: Edward Arnold & Co., 1939

Shlomowitz, R. 'Mortality and the Pacific Labour Trade', *JPH* 22.1/2(1987): 34-55

—— 'Mortality and Indentured Labour in Papua (1885-1941) and New Guinea (1920-1941)', *JPH* 23.1(1988): 70-7

Smith, F.B. *The People's Health 1830-1910.* Canberra: Australian National University Press, 1979

Spidle, J.W. *The German Colonial Civil Service: Organisation, Selection and Training,* PhD Thesis, Stanford University, 1972. Ann Arbour: University Microfilms

Wehler, H.-U. *Bismarck und der Imperialismus.* Cologne and Berlin, 1969

Weindling, P. 'Medicine and Modernization: The Social History of German Health and Medicine', *History of Science* 24(1986): 277-301

—— *Health, Race and German Politics between National Unification and Nazism, 1870-1945.* Cambridge: Cambridge University Press, 1989

Weiss, Sheila. 'The Race Hygiene Movement in Germany', *Osiris,* second series, vol. 3(1987): 193-236

Wigley, S. 'Tuberculosis and New Guinea: historical perspectives, with special reference to the years 1871-1973', in B. G. Burton-Bradley, ed. *A History of Medicine of Papua New Guinea: Vignettes of an earlier Period,* 167-204. Kingsgrove, NSW: Australasian Medical Publishing Co. Ltd., 1990

Winslow, C.E.A. *The conquest of epidemic disease.* Princeton: Princeton University Press, 1944

Worboys, M. 'The Emergence of Tropical Medicine: a study in the establishment of a scientific speciality', in G. Lemaine et al, eds. *Perspectives on the Emergence of Scientific Disciplines,* 75-98. The Hague: Mouton & Co., 1976

Reference works and Bibliographies

Brockhaus' Conversations-Lexikon, thirteenth edition, 1883. Leipzig

Burkill, I.H., ed. *A Dictionary of the Economic Products of the Malay Peninsula.* Kuala Lumpur, 1966

Clasen, U. *Deutsche und deutschstämmige Aerzte in New South Wales und South Australia zwischen 1846 und 1911.* Thesis Dr of Medicine, University of Düsseldorf, 1982

Gillespie, C.C.G., ed. *Dictionary of Scientific Biography.* Vol. 7. New York: Charles Scribner's Sons, 1973

Machlin, L.J., ed. *Handbook of Vitamins.* New York/Basel: Marcel Dekker, 1984

Olpp, G. *Hervorragende Tropenärzte in Wort und Bild.* Munich: Otto Gmelin, 1932

Pagel, J. *Biographisches Lexikon hervorragender Aerzte des neunzehnten Jahrhunderts.* Berlin: Urban & Schwarzenberg, 1901

Schnee, H., ed. *Deutsches Kolonial-Lexikon.* 3 vols. Leipzig, 1920

Sack, P., ed. *German New Guinea: a Bibliography.* Canberra: Australian National University, 1980

Maps and Sketchplan

Maps and sketchplan were prepared by Andrew Davies. The maps are based on maps in Sack & Clark, *German New Guinea: The Annual Reports,* 373-377; the sketchplans on sketches in *Medizinal-Berichte über die Deutschen Schutzgebiete,* 1909/10 and 1911/12.

Index of Persons and Places

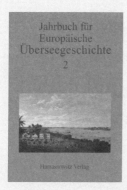

Jahrbuch für Europäische Überseegeschichte 2

Im Auftrag der Forschungsstiftung für Europäische
Überseegeschichte herausgegeben von
M.A. Denzel, H. Gründer, H. Hiery, K. Koschorke,
J. Meier, E. Schmitt, R. Wendt und A. Wirz
2 (2002). 254 Seiten, 6 Abb., br
ISBN 3-447-09282-3
€ 49,– (D) / sFr 84,–

BEITRÄGE

P.C. Emmer, Die europäische Expansion und ihre Folgen im atlantischen Raum,
1500–1800

C. Schnurmann, Die Rekonstruktion eines atlantischen Netzwerkes –
das Beispiel Jakob Leisler, 1660–1691. Ein Editionsprojekt

M. Mann, Von *Khilʿat* zum *Star of India.* Zu Herrschaftslegitimität und Widerstand
in Indien, 1720–1860

M.A. Denzel, Bargeldloser Zahlungsverkehr im europäischen Überseehandel von
der Europäischen Expansion bis zum Ersten Weltkrieg

R. Wendt, Koloniale Metropolen im Bild: Batavia. Erläuterungen zu einem
CD-ROM-Lehrkurs

R.-H. Wippich, Affinität oder Indifferenz in den deutsch-japanischen Beziehungen?
Bemerkungen zur historischen Japanforschung in Deutschland nach 1945

K. Koschorke, Außereuropäische Christentumsgeschichte (Asien, Afrika, Latein-
amerika) – Forschungsstand und Perspektiven einer neuen Disziplin

JUNGES FORUM

C. Pohlmann, Die Auswanderung aus dem Herzogtum Braunschweig im 18. und
19. Jahrhundert im Kräftespiel staatlicher Einflußnahme und öffentlicher Resonanz

W. Fuhrmann, Deutsche Kolonialkinematographie in Afrika: Eine Untersuchung zur
Erforschung des frühen nichtfiktionalen Films

MITTEILUNGEN UND PERSONALIA

REZENSIONEN

HARRASSOWITZ VERLAG · WIESBADEN
www.harrassowitz.de · verlag@harrassowitz.de

Elisabeth Kaske

Bismarcks Missionäre

Deutsche Militärinstrukteure in China 1884–1890

(Asien- und Afrika-Studien der Humboldt-Universität zu Berlin 11)
2002. Ca. 293 Seiten, 8 Abb., gb
ISBN 3-447-04615-5
ca. € 68,– (D) / sFr 116,–

Ausländische Fachkräfte spielten eine Rolle in fast allen chinesischen Reformen zwischen 1870 und 1895, die auf die Selbststärkung des chinesischen Reiches gegen die Bedrohung durch die westlichen Großmächte gerichtet waren. Die Studie relativiert bisherige Forschungen zur Bedeutung von Ausländern im chinesischen Modernisierungsprozess, indem sie einfache Angestellte in chinesischen Diensten in den Mittelpunkt ihrer Betrachtung stellt. Sie untersucht unter zwei Gesichtspunkten eine Gruppe von dreißig ehemaligen deutschen Offizieren und Unteroffizieren, die während des Krieges zwischen China und Frankreich 1884/85 als Militärinstrukteure nach China kamen. Zum einen werden ihre Herkunft, Gründe für das Ausscheiden aus der preußischen Armee bzw. deutschen Marine, Anpassungsstrategien an das Leben in China, der weitere Lebensweg nach dem Ende der Tätigkeit in chinesischen Diensten sowie die eigene Sicht auf China rekonstruiert. Gleichzeitig erörtert Elisabeth Kaske die Arbeitsbedingungen der deutschen Instrukteure in China, die Anforderungen der chinesischen Arbeitgeber an ihre Angestellten und deren Wahrnehmung durch die chinesische Öffentlichkeit, die Rolle der deutschen Diplomaten vor Ort sowie die Bedingungen und Ergebnisse des Transfers von Wissen und Technologien.

HARRASSOWITZ VERLAG · WIESBADEN
www.harrassowitz.de · verlag@harrassowitz.de